THE INVISIBLE SECOND PATIENT

A Dementia Caregiver's Guide To Self-Defence

By Anne-Marie Norman

DISCLAIMER

The Invisible Second Patient is a guide only and does not constitute legal, financial or medical advice. It provides general information that is intended to help those affected by dementia and is up to date at the time of writing in March 2024. If you need legal, financial or medical advice you should consult a professional lawyer, financial adviser or doctor. The Invisible Second Patient was originally written for readers in England and Wales but is available to all.

This book is dedicated to my grandfather,
John Henry Cooper
and my mother, Jane Norman

***

CONTENTS

Help! Someone Give Me A Manual!

How are you? That's right, I said, 'How are YOU?' Not, 'How are your parents, children, aunts, uncles, partner, cat, dog or goldfish?' Just, 'You'. At this point you will have staggered back in shock, and disbelief that someone has actually asked about you, and hopefully you will have landed safely on a soft and comfortable chair. Comfort is what I hope this book will give you.

People like you and I, who look after a loved one with dementia, save the health and social care system about £13 billion every year. Staggering, isn't it? That means you are doing thousands of pounds of unpaid work per year. A live-in carer, employed through an agency costs around the same as a care home; £4,000 a month at time of writing. A professional attorney costs around £100-150 an hour upwards (a law firm's normal hourly rate plus VAT, plus a £300 fee for annual review). But you are not being paid a penny. People may say, 'Oh, but you'll get something in the will', as if that will somehow compensate for the death of your loved one, all the hard work you have done or the fact that you have put your life on hold for so many years. However, in this country there is no law of enforced heirship as there is in France, in other words your parents don't have to leave you anything in their will. Additionally, if the property is used as collateral for care fees then by the time your loved one does pass away there may be no equity left in the property at all.

Do not fall into the trap of thinking that because the government pays carers £80 a week, that is what you are worth. It is not. Remember that you are also emotionally involved and this takes an extra toll on you! The reason I say this is that people who care for elderly relatives with dementia are often under intolerable levels of stress and many are on the point of going bankrupt; they will often be traumatised or financially damaged for years and will rarely get the compensation or support they deserve. Psychologically you may be so worn down that you may even need help with accepting help!

There are about 850,000 people with dementia in the UK at the moment and this figure will keep going up until a cure is found. People with dementia need very high levels of care, most of which is provided informally by family and friends. Dementia caregivers like you tend to be more prone to health issues such as low immunity and heart problems. Many studies have shown that caring for someone with dementia is more stressful than caring for a person who has a physical disability. The large majority of carers in this country are also employed or if they are not, it is because they have had to give up their career in order to be full time carers. Without caregivers like you, people with dementia would need professional help more quickly, and the healthcare system would be overwhelmed. But the support you give comes at a huge cost to your own health and financial wellbeing. Carers of those with dementia are often called the 'invisible second patients' which is why it's the title of this book.

My mother had dementia and I looked after her for five years before she went into a care home. I know what it's like to feel emotionally exhausted and utterly alone. Yes, there are support groups and hubs, but what if you are at work on that day or your loved one refuses to go?

There is a vast amount of information on the internet but you may have to trawl through hundreds of threads to find the answer you need. This is at a time when you are going through extreme stress and are likely to be having your sleep disrupted on a nightly basis. You may also find that much of what is written on the internet is written in a rather dispassionate way; a bit like an essay in which all points of view must be considered. I wanted to get away from that too and write completely from the point of view of a carer. Many of the chat room threads I read seem to berate people who dare to question their role of carer, as if it is a moral duty, not realising the huge strain that it puts on relatives. Unless you have looked after someone with dementia twenty four hours a day, seven days a week for six months at least, you really have no idea what you're talking about and should never judge.

'Am I really a carer?' I hear you ask, surprised that the work you are doing, which is largely taken for granted, is actually a valid job. Well, chances are you are a carer if you do things like helping your loved one to eat, get dressed, shop and attend medical and social appointments. Don't underestimate what you do! Caring isn't just about making sure your loved one takes the right medication or puts on the appropriate clothes, there's the accounting, the form filling, the meetings and the decisions you have to make about end-of-life care. You may end up feeling anxious and depressed or ashamed that you can't do more. You may begin to have entirely unrealistic expectations of yourself. The number of hours you spend caring could be a few hours a day to twenty four hours a day; there's no legal definition of a carer. Some carers live with their elderly relative, some do not. Those who don't live at home have the advantage of having a separate place to stay, those who do will need respite regularly. If you can, keep records of the work that you do as a carer and an attorney (if you are one). You may also find yourself doing repairs on the house your loved one lives in as well as cleaning and coordinating other services. All of this should be recorded and acknowledged.

In this book I will try to give as much useful information as possible to anyone finding themselves in the position of carer. I have focused on the English system although there are similarities between the English, Welsh and Irish systems of social and medical care.

My mother had an excellent mind, having graduated from university with a master's degree. Watching a disease rob her of her talents was heartbreaking. As a child I saw my mother look after her sister, her mother, her father, her husband and her husband's family, as well as holding down a permanent job as a full time teacher. Her whole life was about looking after other people. 'Does that mean I have to do the same?' I thought. The answer is: no, it doesn't. We are a different generation with a different set of challenges. Just because a parent has done it does not mean you have to. But we can still be incredibly proud of what our parents did before us.

I never wanted to be a parent to my parent. Guess what? Mum didn't want me to be her parent either! Your loved one may well refuse to accept this status shift. This is understandable. After all, who wants to relinquish their independence and the authority they have had all their life? Take the situation in which the care agency come round and tell you in no uncertain terms that you can't leave anything sharp or hazardous around the house because these things may be dangerous for your loved one. So you pack up all the scissors, knives, matches, nail files, wall pins and tacks etc. in the house. Your loved one then complains all week about the fact that there are no scissors, or utensils left in the house. Not surprisingly they are frustrated at their belongings being taken away from them. They blame you. They become irate because their authority is being challenged. You end up taking the hit and are caught between a rock and a hard place. You are used to being spoken to in a certain tone of voice and responding in a certain way because you always have. This is just one example of how easily your relationship can become strained. You may have known your elderly relative for half a century or more; it's a very intense relationship and there will sometimes be tension and that is okay. You might not want to feel angry or frustrated but it is not wrong. When you have been dealing with situations like this every day for more than a month, day and night, it starts to grind you down. The mental toll caring takes on your health is huge. This is why you will need respite; the more often the better. Mental exhaustion can extend to your physical health causing sleepless nights, aches and pains, upset stomach and nausea. There is a condition called Carer's Stress Syndrome which is defined as the physical, emotional and mental exhaustion caused by caring for another and this can lead to PTSD. The more you can look after yourself the better.

You will need friends and I mean good friends, not just social media contacts but people around you who will constantly remind you that it's not your fault; it's not your loved one's fault either, it's a disease and you are not responsible for it. Do things that make you happy, make sure you get holidays and days out with friends, go to the gym, date, learn new things. It's not self indulgent. You cannot do it all. You have a right to have a job and a life.

Otherwise you are setting yourself on fire to keep someone else warm. A dementia patient has rights and a carer has rights too. Carers are equally entitled to be safe, physically and psychologically.

This is why it is a good thing to plan your respite as early as possible. Do you have a friend who has a spare room you can borrow occasionally? Sometimes you will feel overwhelmed and it will be unexpected and you won't have time to organise somewhere else to go; you will just need to have a break suddenly. It is a good idea to join a local group or team up with someone in a similar position who lives close by. At the very least you will have someone to swap notes with, you could even swap caring duties; it's often much easier to look after someone who is not related to yourself. It is also useful from the point of view of having someone to back you up when you are having meetings with care staff, social services and so on.

When I was looking after mum there were occasions when I had to get respite by checking into a hotel, while at the same time making sure she had care organised in my absence. Unfortunately Covid often made it more difficult to do this. There were times when you couldn't stay in a hotel or leave your county and this increased the feeling of restriction. On one occasion I did manage to escape to a hotel for a night. I was sitting in the lounge, about to check out. There was only one other guest in the reception area and I heard her chatting to the receptionist. She was saying that she came to the hotel once a month to get respite; her daughter had a disability and this meant that she was her full time carer. But on one sacred weekend a month her partner would look after her daughter so that she could get away.

So there we were, two unpaid carers, both feeling very guilty for leaving our respective relatives but aware on some level that if we didn't do this we wouldn't be around for much longer with the result that our loved ones would have no one to look after them.

On this 'journey' of care you will need a suit of armour, a faithful friend and a cave to hide in. I hope this book is something you can read while you are in that cave. It may not be the manual you expected but I hope it helps, because you deserve help and respect. You need to keep remembering that you are not selfish and you are not alone. Whatever anyone else tells you, you are a wonderful, kind and selfless human being.

How Dementia In Others Affects You

There are two behaviours associated with dementia that most people find particularly challenging. One is continuous repetition and the other is wandering.

<u>Repetition</u>

Hearing the constant repetition of the same phrase or question is mentally tortuous. Your loved one with dementia may repeat the same phrase fifty times a day or more. They may say, 'Have you turned the light off?' or, 'Have you fed the cat?' You will reply, 'Yes, I have'. A minute later they will ask the same question and again you will reply that you have done what they asked. You will remain patient, knowing that they probably need reassurance and may be anxious; this anxiety and loss of short-term memory is not their fault but a symptom of the disease. When they have been repeating the same thing for about an hour your ability to cope with it will wane. It will feel as if someone is scraping a piece of chalk down a blackboard. This can be extremely distressing and can cause what is known as 'cognitive fatigue'. It is not normal for our brains to be perpetually processing the same information. The result of this constant repetition on you is that you may find it harder to retain information or concentrate. You can end up feeling as if you have been fighting a battle all day. Sometimes your relative may, if they are still using the phone, phone you incessantly. The first time they call you may be happy to chat and respond as normal, even if you have to repeat yourself several times, the second time they call you may be slightly irritated, particularly if you are at work or looking after a child. The third time you may tactfully say to your loved one that they have just called and remind them that you are busy. The fourth time you may just have to ignore the call, otherwise you will be on the phone all day talking about buying cat food from the supermarket. Incessant calls at night can prevent you from getting a good night's sleep. Sometimes it can help to write things down on a white board and put it in a prominent place in the house. That way you can point it out when your loved one asks. Sometimes this works and sometimes it doesn't as they may still ask the question or ask a different one such as, 'Where is the white board?'

If you are someone who suffers from anxiety, depression or migraines all this repetition can worsen your symptoms. Some people who suffer from migraines get something called 'hyperacuesis' which means they are hypersensitive to noises. After having a migraine their hearing goes back to normal, but you can imagine how devastating this can be if you are already under stress and someone is constantly trying to get your attention by talking, shouting or screaming. Some people, me included, are just naturally highly sensitive to sound, smell, light and so on. Listening to the incessant crying of a baby can be a form of torture for some people; apparently it does affect the nervous systems of mothers, whereas others do not mind it at all. Auditory repetition is used in interrogations as a technique to break someone down. Sometimes it is made deliberately worse by the illogicality of the questions which are designed to disorientate someone. So imagine this on a daily basis for the duration of your waking hours. A carer looking after someone with dementia can find themselves in this very challenging position.

Have you ever become irritated by the sound of a dinner companion scraping their fork on a plate or a passenger on a bus behind you noisily chewing gum? There's a condition called misophonia and people who have it are not just irritated by certain sounds, they find them completely intolerable. Certain sounds act as triggers for an involuntary physical and emotional reflex in the body of the person who has it. The sound sets off the autonomic nervous system, which is linked to emotion. A person who has misophonia will react every time to the sound, whether they want to or not. If you have a condition such as this it is unlikely you will be able to tolerate living with someone with dementia. Obviously, there are certain therapies such as cognitive behavioural therapy which can help to a certain extent but the reason I mention this condition is because it shows how hearing the same repetitive sounds can negatively affect a person's nervous system. Some people are much more sensitive to sound than others and will actually feel pain when they hear loud noise. So it's not surprising that carers, who have to listen to shouting, screaming and repetitive speech can become burnt out or depressed.

When I raised this issue with professionals during my carer's assessment they didn't seem to feel it was really serious and it wasn't properly addressed. So what can you do about it when you are left on your own with it? Use noise cancelling headphones? But then how would you be able to hear your loved one call for help if they needed it? The best option in my opinion, apart from respite, is to have your loved one looked after in a care home setting with a team of people to look after them. In this way, the caring duties will be shared and caring for someone with dementia is arguably easier when you are not personally connected to the patient. But of course this is very expensive if you can't get help from the NHS or local authority and few of us can afford to pay out £5,000 a month from our own personal funds.

Distraction is a technique that can be used but this requires a lot of energy. The person with dementia may not wish to engage in the distraction. So you may say, 'Let's watch the weather on TV'. They may reply that they don't want to and then a few minutes later resume the same questions. Or they may simply say 'no' to everything you suggest. The constant questioning, from their point of view, is probably because they are seeking comfort and reassurance, they need to know you are there for them and this is completely understandable because they want normality and a sense of control. It must be agonising to feel helpless in this way and to be vaguely aware that you are losing your ability to make sense of the world. It is the disease that is causing them to feel this, it is not who they really are. Memory aids can help to a certain extent. For example, the whiteboard mentioned above, large clocks and calendars which show in the dark or electronic devices that tell someone when to take their medicine. The repetition could also be because there is something your loved one is trying to communicate. Are they cold because a window is open, for example? If they are, closing the window could help.

What made your loved one happy? Joyful experiences can lessen anxiety. In the early stages of dementia mum used to like doing jigsaw puzzles of places she had visited abroad and we also had puzzles made from photographs of the family. She found listening to music comforting but did not want a radio, television or any kind of technology in her room; possibly due to the complexity of technology and a sense that she was not in control of it because her mind could no longer grasp it. At later stages of dementia she enjoyed having animals around. One of the gifts she received was a robotic companion cat complete with fur! This was especially designed for those with dementia and mum seemed to find it very beneficial.

So there are many things that can help but you will need respite on a regular basis from the incessant questioning. Do not feel guilty for not having a solution, you may as well feel guilty for not having a cure for the common cold! You are doing your best in the face of a very cruel disease.

<u>Wandering</u>

Wandering is also known as elopement. Sounds romantic? It's not. It is another quite harrowing aspect of dementia. It is defined as 'leaving one's dwelling unescorted'. Elopement can happen at home or in a care home, even in the early stages of dementia. Wandering can increase the risk of injury, accidents and hypothermia or hyperthermia. This can put a huge burden on you. You can end up feeling exasperated as you try to keep tabs on your loved one while at the same time being unable to restrict them. It can also open you up to some quite unpleasant reactions from neighbours and other people in your area who may call the police or paramedics and make you feel as if you are at the centre of some kind of criminal investigation. You may start to receive calls from various people telling you that your elderly relative is 'roaming the streets' and that 'someone' (that would be you, of course) has to take responsibility for them! Whilst you can buy carpet sensors and GPS trackers there is always the possibility that your loved one will refuse to wear the GPS pendant or watch or will not take the handbag you have hidden it in, or that they will avoid the carpet sensor or throw it out. A fall alarm can be useful or can cause more problems than it solves. Perhaps they are worth a try but everyone is an individual and dementia affects people in different ways so what works for one person may not work for another.

It is all very well for people to say that you shouldn't 'let' your elderly relative out. It is nearly impossible to stop them and it is also illegal unless you have what is called a DoLS (Deprivation of Liberty Safeguarding order) in place. Don't feel bad if you didn't know that. Not many people do. You were probably just trying your best to keep your parent safe by keeping them inside. (I'll talk more about DoLS in a later chapter). The chances are that you are well aware of the risks and have been battling with your mother or father for years trying to get them to listen to you. You may have asked your parent or relative to stop standing on chairs or pleaded with them to refrain from going out driving at night. You may then have been faced with a barrage of rudeness, aggression and ridicule that will eventually have reduced you to tears, not once a day, but several times a day. Dementia is extremely difficult to predict. Therefore, there is no way that you can know what your loved one is going to do next. You don't have a crystal ball. It will be very difficult for you, as the person looking after them to know at what point they should stop going for walks alone. They may never have been lost, injured or mugged before. Then one day it happens. A person with dementia can have varying capacity and what they might be able to do one day, they won't be able to do the next.

Let's say one day you are at home and you hear a car pull up outside. It's one of your parent's friends and lo and behold, your parent is sitting beside them in the passenger seat. Your loved one has been escorted home because she or he has been walking around looking lost and disorientated but once inside they tell you not to disclose this to anyone else. This could be a good opportunity to involve a third party for your own and your loved one's protection. For example, you could contact the adult social services department of your local council. They have a duty to do a free needs assessment under the Care Act 2014. You can book this online even if your loved one isn't eligible for state funded care at the time and you are in work. As you and I know this could turn into another problem for you. Your loved one will never want to be dependant on you or anyone else; they will want to hang onto their independence for as long as possible, but it is a hard thing to get used to after a lifetime of listening to them telling you what to do. You may suddenly feel like you are 'going behind their back' and telling on them. I had a conversation with mum, saying that it was really up to her but there was no harm in seeing the local authority as they may be able to suggest helpful adaptations. Eventually she agreed. After mum had her assessment I was asked if I wanted a carer's assessment as well. I said that I did, so an assessor came to our home and talked to me for about an hour. I completed a 'Caregiver's Strain Index' questionnaire and I talked to the assessor about the difficulties I faced in keeping mum safe. However, to be honest, I didn't find this very helpful. The assessor couldn't give me any advice about the behavioural problems associated with dementia. She suggested that I contact a local dementia hub. I did so but unfortunately mum did not want to go there, even for a cup of coffee (again, this was solely due to the disease; mum had always been a very sociable person before she suffered from dementia). There was a relatives group who got together once a week but the meetings were always at times when I was at work so it wasn't possible to go.

The other issue is that in order to go to any face to face meetings you will have to get care for your loved one in your absence. Emergency respite was suggested to me but only because I might be ill and then there would be no one to look after mum, not because I might desperately need some time off for myself. I was given a leaflet about contingency planning. You have to fill in a form, carry a Carer's Card and let your GP know (more forms for you to fill in). However, there was no one who would agree to help out in an emergency or be listed as a contact on the form.

The other issue with the Carer's Assessment is that things can very quickly take a downturn when it comes to dementia so while one week everything could be fine (that's of course the week when they will visit you) the next you have a crisis on your hands. It is the variability of the disease and the unpredictability of it which makes living with it so hard. You may have carers support organisations in your area though I did find that they were sometimes slow to respond, often taking more than a week to answer by email. Once again, it is all very well getting support in place when you need respite, but your loved one may decide that they are not going to accept any help. You could join a dementia forum or Facebook page; these can be quite comforting as you share your experiences with other people and realise that you are not alone. Online communities have the advantage that you can post and receive answers at any time of day or night.

Can social services force someone into a care home even if they don't want to go? The answer is yes, they can but only if the person's care needs are not being met at home. Being forced into a care home should only be done as a last resort and it should be carried out in a way which is least upsetting for all concerned. The emphasis should be on making your loved one feel as safe and comfortable as possible in their new home, with lots of familiar things around them. Many care homes now integrate therapies and social events throughout the week into the schedule of care and are no longer lonely or sad places. A care home may well be preferable to your loved one spending most of the day on their own or with only one other person.

Can care and assistance be forced on your loved one? Someone can only be force fed or forced to have certain treatment in limited circumstances. The relevant legislation is found in the Mental Capacity Act 2005, The Mental Health Act 1983 and by looking at any advanced decision (living will) or Lasting Power of Attorney that the person has made. If there is any uncertainty the case can be referred to court but whatever decision is made it must always be in the patient's best interests.

Duty of care

What is a duty of care? It's a legal duty anyone can have towards anyone else but it usually arises when one individual or group does something which could potentially harm someone else or themselves physically, mentally, or financially. Essentially, it's about not harming other people. You won't find it in a statute because it's part of the common law (the principles of law that have developed over centuries). An activity which may harm someone includes driving a car, giving bad financial advice or serving contaminated food. When a breach of a duty of care has taken place it's called negligence. But to be negligent the harm must be what is called 'reasonably foreseeable' (a legal term meaning you could have predicted it), a close relationship must exist and it must be fair to make someone liable. Take the following example: It's the middle of winter and a biker hits some ice, loses control and swerves into the forecourt of a restaurant, hitting a ten foot tall fast food sign shaped like a lobster. He gets injured and bruises his face where the lobster claw hit him and says the restaurant are negligent for placing the sign there. Are the restaurant negligent? Probably not. It was so unlikely to happen that it couldn't have been foreseeable; the bad road conditions contributed to it and caused the chain of events.

The reason I mention duty of care is that it comes into play when we are placed in the position of looking after someone else, particularly when they are elderly or frail and we are in close proximity to them. So what does that mean for you? Are you supposed to escort your parents everywhere all the time? No you're not, unless you are a professional carer and they are your patient. If you are a professional the duty of care is higher than if you are not. There is no legal duty to volunteer to help in an emergency situation either. Even if a nurse, for example, is present at a road traffic accident they do not have an automatic duty of care to give medical help to any person injured in the accident. This is because nurses do not always have the kind of training which could help the injured person. If you are at the scene of an accident and you are trying to help but are not a doctor or nurse, make that clear by letting others know. If you are at home or out with your loved one and they have an accident you would be expected to stay with them and call for help as soon as possible by phoning the emergency services. Your duty of care in that case would be to try to keep your parent free from further harm, and make them as comfortable as possible in the circumstances while professional help arrived. But you are not expected to be present with them at all times or to be able to protect them from every possible hazard. You cannot be everywhere all at once!

Sundowning – what is it?
Sometimes your loved one's symptoms may get worse at night. This is known as sundowning. This can make your, and their, sleep schedule irregular and may cause a great deal of extra stress as you try to keep track of their waking and sleeping habits. You may be woken up at night by your loved one who is unable to sleep and may be behaving strangely; tearing up papers, rearranging their belongings or doing gardening in the middle of the night.

Escape room – how do I get out of here?
Sometimes respite is as simple as taking a walk or calling a friend and sometimes it means going on holiday for a week or two. Of course, you have to make sure your loved one is being looked after by someone capable of doing so. This is frustrating and limits your freedom as you not only have to plan the trip but also your loved one's replacement care for the time you are away, so it takes a lot more time and effort than simply booking a flight and hotel.

In terms of getting respite for yourself, another strategy is having a friend who has a spare room they can let you borrow when things get too much. If you're lucky enough to have an outside office or cabin then that's a really good way to be 'together' yet apart. If you can afford it you could get a caravanette or a mobile home. Anywhere that gives you a bit of privacy and your own toilet and washbasin is going to be a good idea when you are living with someone who is incontinent. Another idea is being paid to house sit for people who are away on holiday. Look for websites that say, 'House Sitting Jobs', you will have to sign up and provide paperwork for obvious reasons but it can be a good way of spending time away from home for free.

If you do want to go on holiday with your loved one you still can. There are hotels and guest houses which cater for people with dementia. All you have to do is give them a ring or send an email and they will let you know if they are able to cater for you both. You could go on a day trip first, not too far away, to see how well your relative copes, then you can get home quickly should they become anxious and insist on going home. You could take some things that your loved one is familiar with such as a favourite blanket or clothes; these items may help make them feel secure. When you have no control over changes to your body and mind you reach for whatever gives you a sense of continuity and normality. For someone with dementia visiting a past holiday destination or a place they used to live could also give them a lot of pleasure.

Scapegoats and other animals (how families change)
Dementia can change family dynamics dramatically. Even the closest relationships can suffer under the weight of financial tensions and it is interesting how the mention of one word: 'money' can cause deep seated rifts. Legal arrangements can be complex. Years of one sibling caring for a parent can cause resentment when the other siblings may be working hard and may feel that it isn't their job. Arguments and tensions can surface often. Does one sibling believe the parent loved the other one more? Did one child get more attention? All of this can resurface when dealing with an elderly parent.

If your loved one has been married more than once and you have half siblings it is more likely that disputes can arise about financial and legal issues. Know that this is the norm rather than the exception and that it will pass. No one's family is perfect. There is no standard you have to live up to. You just have to do what feels right for you. Just because we have DNA in common with someone doesn't mean we have to be their best buddy.

Social distancing takes on a whole new meaning when you are caring for someone who has double incontinence and the fact that you can no longer invite friends and family round isolates you more. So you may find yourself alone and feeling that you have been 'left to do all the caring' by your family. How do you manage such a situation? You could try the informal route; talk to them and hope that they will respond in a reasonable way. Or you could get family or friends to mediate informally. An uncle, aunt or cousin could help with mediation in some circumstances if you really can't, or even a trusted family friend, although sometimes you may find they won't because they are afraid of 'interfering'. If all else fails you can choose professional mediation. The costs will be about £100-£150 per hour. There are also mediators who specialise in will disputes. The very last resort is to let the Court of Protection take over but this is to be avoided if you can as it is very expensive and some would say equally upsetting and intrusive.

Your elderly relative may try to exert control over you (consciously or subconsciously) by contacting other siblings and playing you off against each other, telling them how horrible you have been. How very dare you upset mother? You may find yourself playing out the old family dynamics with your siblings who may make you feel as if you've gone back in time to your school days. From child to parent back to child again; your status may change by the hour! Your parent may accuse you of being the worst son or daughter in the world or try to manipulate you by saying things like, 'I feel like a burden now', 'I don't want to be on my own','You don't care about me at all!' Well, if that's the case join the club, there are thousands of 'bad children' all around the globe!

What about the young children in the family? How do you talk to them about dementia? For a child, seeing their grandparent, great aunt or uncle getting old, forgetful and possibly aggressive can be very unsettling and cause anxiety. Children pick up immediately on the tiniest display of fear from adults. A child may be confused as to why grandma or grandpa is not engaging with them in the same way anymore or has been taken away from them. You can let them know that they haven't done anything wrong and grandma is not angry with them. They may pick up on all the upset and emotion that is going on in the family. 'Why can't anyone make grandma better?' they may ask. There are many good children's books about dementia which explain the disease in a way that is easy for children to understand. You can read these with your child or niece/nephew and use it as a way of talking about the subject. This will help you to explain dementia to them. You can say it is a disease that affects the brain and it makes people forgetful. They may be afraid that the same thing is going to happen to their parents, or to them. There are lots of activities such as drawing, writing, and music that children can use to express themselves and these are also helpful in connecting with their elderly relative who may also love singing, for example.

<u>**Anticipatory grief**</u>

Now this is what I call a strange animal. I had never experienced it before. I had experienced normal grief; the kind where someone dies and you feel it afterwards, like a slow tidal wave of immense sadness, but I had never experienced the loss of a person before death. Dementia, as we all know, is called, 'The Long Goodbye'. It is a slow loss over many years. You may find yourself grieving in stages. The first time your loved one starts repeating the same phrases, you may experience a wave of sadness, then once again when you are told their going into care is 'an option', or when eventually they look at you as if they don't know who you are. It's an incremental loss. It can put you in a state of emotional limbo, in between life and death. You can feel unable to move forward because the impending final loss could be coming tomorrow or in ten years from now. It can get to the stage where, every time the care home phones, you are expecting the worst. This is a difficult thing to go through when it happens again and again over a period of years.

How to deal with anticipatory grief? There are many therapies and support groups for people who are facing death in one way or another (I mention some of them in the chapter about the end of life later in the book). Depending on your beliefs you could join a group that is spiritual or in which you can express your feelings through art or writing, for example. There are some excellent videos on YouTube and other social media about how to cope when you are going through this experience.

Prepare And Protect Yourself

Knowledge is power. Sounds dramatic, but it is!

The legal framework
The fact is that people are not obligated to provide personal or financial care for their elderly parents. The law says that elderly care is the responsibility of the NHS and/or local authorities.

In England the government's decisions flow down to the Secretary of State for Health and Social Care then to the Department of Health and Social Care, NHS England and the Care Quality Commission. The Welsh NHS is separate from the English NHS as Wales has its own devolved government which oversees both health and social care.

The local council's social care budget comes from a lump sum from central government as well as council tax whereas the NHS is funded mainly from general taxes and national insurance. Apparently in years gone by people thought that the NHS budget would reduce with time as the health of the nation improved! That would have been lovely, wouldn't it? But unfortunately, that has not happened because people are now living longer. I have recently heard that ninety is the new eighty.

You will find the legal framework for the NHS in the NHS Constitution for England and in case law, EU law and common law. The way the NHS works is not streamlined and is not the single entity that most people imagine it is. Just one action that a nurse or doctor takes can be covered by various sources of law, legal obligations, regulations and duties, that's not including moral sentiments or cultural factors. Codes of ethics don't cover every situation. There are various National Health Service Acts, the latest one being the 2006 Act. Not surprisingly the law relating to healthcare and medicine changes frequently as new drugs and technology become available and society changes (which is why medical staff have to do so many continuing professional development courses). The legal framework for the social care of adults in the UK is currently The Care Act 2014 and this includes assessment and safeguarding. The law of the NHS is fragmented and difficult to negotiate.

The difference between social care and healthcare can be important when you are applying for funding (see the chapter entitled 'Funding'). Social care is about helping people to stay independent, improving their ability to interact socially and protecting people from situations such as abuse. It includes assessments and local authority funding for care home places. Healthcare, on the other hand, is focused on the treatment, control and prevention of a disease (such as dementia), illness, injury or disability and the care or aftercare of a person with these issues. This includes NHS continuing healthcare funding and medication.

The previous government had been talking about making changes to the funding of care. These changes were planned to have taken effect from October 2025. This would have meant that no one in England would have had to pay more than £86,000 for their care during their lifetime, Unfortunately, even if this is implemented in 2025, the rule will not be retrospective so you will not be able to say, 'I have already paid £20,000 for my own care therefore from October 2025 I should only have to pay another £66,000 and no more'; your self funding contributions will be calculated from October 2025 onward. Let's keep our fingers crossed that funding does improve with successive governments.

The Mental Capacity Act 2005
This is the Act that established the Office of the Public Guardian and the new Lasting Powers of Attorney which replaced the old style Enduring Powers of Attorney. The main idea behind the Mental Capacity Act is that people should be allowed to make their own decisions when they can. If someone has an LPA (Lasting Power of Attorney) the attorney can make decisions for the donor (the donor is the person who made the LPA). If the donor really doesn't have mental capacity the attorney/attorneys can make decisions for them but it always has to be in the best interests of the donor. However, as carers know, mental capacity can vary and the problem with dementia is that it is difficult to know when someone is going to be without capacity and when they are going to be with capacity; what day are we talking about, Monday or Saturday? Are we talking morning or evening or in the middle of the night? How can my loved one talk lucidly about one topic but not another? People can lack mental capacity due to an accident for example and then recover but who knows when and how much? There is still much to be worked out in terms of creating legal clarity for carers.

Safeguarding
Safeguarding laws seek to protect adults who can't protect themselves because they have a need for care and support, even if the local authority doesn't meet those needs. A local authority must promote wellbeing in everything it does.

Safeguarding is mostly governed by The Care Act 2014 although The Human Rights Act 1998 also plays a part. Under Section 42 of the Care Act, local authorities have a duty to make enquiries if they think an adult with care needs is being abused or is at risk of harm. A social worker or health professional can carry out an investigation into what has happened. It could be something like a resident in a care home not getting the medicines they need or it could be a person with dementia being scammed. Abuse or neglect could be many different things and it's not limited to a list as every case is unique.

When abuse is suspected, an enquiry can be carried out by a social worker or a health professional. If a crime has been committed, this will be carried out by the police. If the enquiry is carried out by a social worker they may decide that someone needs to visit the person at risk, or phone calls need to be made.

How to raise a safeguarding concern

Who can raise a concern? Anyone; a friend, relative, neighbour or professional carer and you can too. You can raise a safeguarding concern by filling in a form online on your local authority website or by calling them. A social worker from the council will respond to you and make a plan with other health professionals and the police as to how they can find out more about the abuse and hopefully stop it as soon as possible. This is called an enquiry. The local authority must 'make enquiries' where there is 'reasonable cause' to suspect an adult with care needs is being abused. Try to talk to your elderly relative before you do this, there is a part of the form which asks if they are aware that it has been submitted. If they have dementia at any stage, they may forget your conversation quickly but you can record the fact that you have spoken to them and what you both said in a note. You can also, if you wish, report a safeguarding concern anonymously.

What if someone reports me to safeguarding?

Unfortunately, there are some very spiteful people out there who, because they have nothing better to do or because they don't want to take on a responsibility they are supposed to have, will try and blame you for the fact that your relative is wandering or not looking after themselves. The chances are that you will already have had hundreds of sleepless nights trying to keep an eye on your loved one to no avail, as well as countless arguments in an attempt to stop them doing things that may pose a risk to themselves or others (such as riding a bike or going up ladders). Needless to say whoever has reported you has not seen all of this take place and has never been in this situation themselves. Sometimes a person with dementia can have hallucinations or delusions which may cause them to blame you for something you haven't done. Hallucinations are usually either visual or auditory. It's very rare that they are multisensory.

What sort of things could happen? A person with dementia could hallucinate that a person is turning into an animal, or that there are insects all over the floor. They could become paranoid and believe that you are their enemy when you have done nothing but be kind to them.

It may feel odd having someone telling you how to treat your mother. It can feel (and did feel for me) as if someone is intruding on one of the closest and most special relationships you can have in your life; that of mother and child. Remember you have rights. You have the right to challenge anything that is said about you.

You have the right to read all information about you which is kept by social services and the police. You have the right not to be blamed for something that could never be your fault. Anybody making a false accusation against you can be charged and convicted for wasting police time. Alternatively, they might be charged with perverting the course of justice which is more serious.

If you are reported to safeguarding, social services will call asking what has happened. You will then be able to give your side of the story. The social worker will then decide if any further action needs to be taken. If someone such as a neighbour has falsely said something about you which has been recorded for example, to the police, social services or a GP, you have every right to obtain the records in which you are mentioned. If authorities are having meetings that you are not invited to you have a right to read what was discussed. You deserve to be consulted by social services politely and by letter or email addressed to you. You can't be expected to be answering calls all day while you are also attending meetings at work, doing your job, taking your child to the doctor or driving. Social services may be so overstretched that they may not always be able to speak to you immediately or directly but there should be some way of communicating with them which is effective.

Once you find out what has been said about you, you can decide whether or not it is correct. The Information Commissioner's Office website is a good place to start for information on this topic. If the information is not accurate you can apply to get it corrected. Everyone has the right to rectification if authorities hold inaccurate factual information about them and keeping inaccurate information about someone is a breach of UK GDPR. If this happens to you with any government body let them know. The public body must respond to the request within a reasonable time and not delay. They should give an answer at the latest within one month from the first day after the request was received. They must then let you know in writing whether you can have access to the information or not and if not, the reasons why. Additionally, they must tell you how you can raise a complaint against them if you want to (this will be through the Information Commissioner's Office or a court).

Remember that you also have rights against public authorities under Article 8 of The Human Rights Act 1998, which is the right to respect for private and family life, home and correspondence. Records that are held about you by social services will normally be held for only six years. After that time they must be destroyed securely.

It's important that you get some help and support during a time like this. If you are caring for someone who is hallucinating it can be very frightening for you too and you could end up doubting your own sanity. I remember mum saying she could hear the doorbell ring and I wondered, 'Did it really ring? Did I not hear it? Have I got a problem with my hearing?' I think we are so conditioned to respond to our parents in a particular way because they have been the voice of reason for so long that it is quite a shock when that changes. Medications can help your loved one with hallucinations so you could ask for a medication review from the GP. It may also help to rule out urinary tract or other infections as these can be a cause of hallucinations.

Self-neglect

Unintentional self-neglect is a difficult thing to deal with due to the human rights element. There's a limit to what the law can do if an elderly person decides to live in a particular way. Self-neglect includes not looking after your own hygiene, health, or surroundings. Whether or not safeguarding will need to be put in place depends on how well the person can control their own behaviour. Social services will tend to make decisions on a case by case basis as every individual is different. So if your loved on is not looking after themselves, not washing properly, hoarding or not eating healthily, you could let the local authority adult social care team know as they may be able to offer help. They will carry out an assessment and try to engage the person and work with them to make improvements.

Financial abuse

Financial and economic abuse includes having money or property stolen and being 'scammed'. This is becoming increasingly common with the rise of online fraud. I have even found that despite putting stickers on the door saying, 'No cold callers' they still call! Possibly because they think that the stickers mean a vulnerable person is living in the house. I am talking about people like rogue builders who tell you they can see things wrong with your roof, fencing or pathway. This is one reason why having an LPA for Finance and Property is a good idea. Neighbourhood Watch schemes can also help, particularly in keeping an eye on potential scammers in your area on a day to day basis.

If you see your loved one has a lack of clothing or food or an inability to pay bills this could be a red flag. Other indicators include unexplained withdrawals from an account or sudden or unexpected changes in a will or other financial documents. Talking of documents, keep an eye on them. Long before your loved one begins to suffer from dementia you could try to organise important documents and streamline their filing. I know it's hard work but it could make things much easier at a later stage; you won't have so much to do then and it won't be so overwhelming. I spent months shredding paperwork that was out of date and irrelevant. I also sorted and filed the important documents so I knew where the bank statements were, the accounts, what was in them and how to access them. This was a job and a half. I colour coded, yes I am a colour coder! I made spreadsheets and I bought dividers and folders for all the receipts I would need to keep as an attorney. Do whatever works best for you and don't worry about your relative querying it. If you have power of attorney you will need to organise paperwork and you may find that the one you care for is actually grateful that it's a job they don't have to do any more. More on scams and how to avoid them later.

Domestic abuse

This is abuse that occurs within a domestic environment. It includes violence, psychological, sexual, financial, and emotional abuse. The Domestic Abuse Act 2021 deals with abuse between people who are personally connected, such as family members. There are other criminal offences which relate to abuse by care staff, sales people, or health and housing professionals who may come into contact with you or your loved one, for example, fraud offences. Withholding things like medication, food or heating is an offence, as is not giving access to hearing aids, dentures, or other equipment that someone relies on for their everyday healthcare.

The Human Rights Act 1998 includes a right not to be tortured, or treated in an inhuman or degrading way (this is Article 3). So abuse and neglect can also be a violation of Article 3.

Can a person be removed from their own home?

If a local authority thinks someone living at home is being abused or neglected, they normally don't have the automatic power to come and take the person away. However, if the person has the capacity and wants to leave they can be helped to get to a safe place while an investigation is carried out. If the vulnerable person lacks mental capacity the local authority needs to work out what is in the person's best interests and try to manage any risk to their wellbeing. Obviously, they need to find out whether or not the person has a Lasting Power Of Attorney (LPA) or a deputy authorised to make decisions, otherwise they may have to apply to the Court of Protection to take the person to a place of safety. If family and friends disagree about where the person lacking capacity should live, an application can be made to the Court of Protection and they (the court) has to decide. If you are affected by the above situation, it may be a good idea to get specialist legal advice. You can go online and look for Court of Protection lawyers but always make sure that they are registered with the Solicitors Regulation Authority and are on the Law Society Website. Also, check that they have insurance.

Property And What To Do With It

Before your loved one's dementia has progressed too far they can transfer their property to you but there are caveats. There is an inheritance tax issue and also an issue around care home fees.

In terms of inheritance tax, if a person gifts a house to their child this is called a 'potentially exempt transfer' which means it might be exempt from inheritance tax but it might not be, depending on when the person who is doing the gifting dies. A potentially exempt transfer is also called a PET for short. So if the person dies within seven years of gifting the property then it is going to be included in the inheritance tax calculation (how much tax is paid depends on how soon the person dies). But if the person survives for seven years after gifting the property there won't be inheritance tax to pay. Once the person has given the property away they won't be able to live in it or stay in it for any length of time or get rent from it, otherwise the house would be considered part of their estate even if they survive for more than seven years afterwards. (Though they would be able to stay for short social visits, of course). The reason for this is that they will be seen as still getting a benefit from it. They could pay rent to their children but it would have to be market rent and their children would have to include it in their income for income tax purposes.

Another issue is that if someone gives their house to their children they could be forced out of the house if their children want to rent or sell the property or live there themselves. If the children get married and then get divorced then who knows where the property may end up; it could go to their child's ex spouse! Additionally, if their son or daughter were to get into debt and ended up bankrupt, the property would form part of their estate which could then be claimed by creditors wanting to get their money back. The courts will be able to make decisions about the property without the permission of the previous owner. The most unthinkable situation would be where the person gifting the property outlives their child/children who they have given the house to. The property could then go to that child's spouse or whoever their beneficiaries are. This is why a lot of lawyers hesitate to advise their elderly clients to sign their houses over to their children. It may not be in their client's best interests because family dynamics change all the time. When gifting a property the giver should also think about the potential capital gains tax (CGT) bill. This happens when a person is not living in the house and it goes up in value or if it's a second home that you are giving away. The CGT payable would be on the increase in value between the time you first bought it and the time when you gave it away.

If your parent wants to give their property to you they should get legal advice; a local solicitor should be able to do this. The reason is that the local authority could see the gift as a 'deliberate deprivation of assets'. In other words, you are deliberately giving everything away so that you won't have to pay care fees. This will surface during the financial assessment that the local authority carry out when you ask for help with care home fees. If this is found to be the case, the local authority has the power to reverse the transfer of ownership so the house ownership will go back to the parent/s and the local authority will take it into consideration when calculating assistance with care home fees.

These are all things your loved one needs to think about before signing over the house to you or someone else and of course they have to have mental capacity when they do it. It is better to be aware of these things far in advance so that you can plan accordingly.

<u>Tenancy in common</u>

What is a severed tenancy when it's at home? Severed ... Sounds nasty, doesn't it? But it could be very useful to you. If your parents own their own home and they want you to get the benefit of it when they are no longer around, having a tenancy in common could help. There are two main types of home ownership in England and Wales: they are called 'Joint Tenancy' and 'Tenancy in Common'. If your parents own their home as joint tenants this means they own the house together as a whole. In other words, they own both the legal title and the equitable title equally. It's a bit of a strange expression as the use of the word 'tenancy' makes you think it's to do with a rental situation which it isn't. In English and Welsh law currently you can't completely split the legal and equitable title to a property but the next best thing you can do is to split (sever) the equitable ownership. What this means is that when you come to sell the house, you will both get the net proceeds of sale that reflect the percentage ownership you have. For example if the 'tenancy' is split 50/50 and the net proceeds of sale of the property are £600,000 then one party will get £300,000 and the other will get £300,000.

How is this helpful to you? If your parents split the 'tenancy' and become 'tenants in common' that means that they can put their half of the property into their will and leave their half to whoever they want. So they can leave their half of the property to you and/or your siblings. When one parent dies their half will then go to those beneficiaries. The other half will still be owned by the other parent who can continue living in the house. When that parent goes into care the local authority will only be able to take into account that parent's percentage ownership of the house. What then is the value of the house? Does it, in fact, have any real value at all? After all, who wants to buy a house that is partly owned by one or two other people? It could be argued that the value of the property is therefore zero. It could then be argued that the person about to go into care does not own a property of any value and the local authority can't take the house into account in their care funding calculations.

<u>The will and preparations</u>
Does it help to have a will? In short, yes, it does. Even if you have an estate worth less than £5,000 it still helps to have a will. Why? Because what you are aiming for is to have no ambiguity; zero, zilch, de nada. Should the executors be told who they are? Yes, definitely. Should there be any surprises or secret trusts? Preferably not. Should you leave mysterious letters, packages and films with you as the star of the show from beyond the grave? No. So if you can, and I know it's really hard, talk to your parents about their wills before dementia takes hold.

There are currently proposals to reform the law of will-making and you can find information about this on the Law Society's website. The Wills Act, which came into effect in 1837, was made rather a long time ago and wills are being disputed more and more frequently so it was thought a good idea to update the law. Proposals include updating the formalities for making a will, looking at the validity of electronic wills and changing the test for capacity to make a will (obviously this is due to the large numbers of people now living with dementia). A person with dementia can still make a will if they understand what they are doing. Sounds complicated? It is. There are of course legal provisions one can point to. But how can someone such as a lawyer accurately judge capacity when they have only just met someone? Often it is left to a doctor to do this but again, I think it is highly complex as dementia is not necessarily a linear or predictable disease.

Can a will be changed after death?

Yes, in certain circumstances. The beneficiaries, if all in agreement, can do what is called a Deed of Variation which varies the terms of the Will (i.e. who gets what) after death. If you wish to do this you can go and see a solicitor who can draw up the Deed for you. The cost will be around £1,000.

Certain relatives and dependants have a right to challenge a will, or the rules of intestacy, by making a claim under the Inheritance (Provision for Family and Dependants) Act 1975. There are time limits though so if you want to do this you should start the ball rolling as soon as possible after the person dies. At the least within six months after obtaining the grant of probate or letters of administration (letters of administration are what you need when someone dies without a will or executors). In the UK an individual can give away their estate according to their wishes but in some other countries, there is a law of forced heirship. This means that a person must leave a certain percentage of their estate to their children. (which is possibly why DNA tests are not encouraged by the French!).

In terms of the Inheritance (Provision for Family and Dependants) Act 1975 the classes of applicant who can bring a claim include: a child of the deceased or a person who was treated as a child of the family by the deceased, among others. The process is likely to take a few years and the cost will be as per the solicitor's hourly rate. Legal costs can run into tens of thousands of pounds but generally, if you win, the loser will pay those costs. You can possibly pay via a Conditional Fee Agreement ("CFA"), or insurance or a litigation loan. However, it is a lengthy, emotional and financially draining experience. It may result in an agreement pre-court which could be a better solution for you. In any case get good advice before you sign any type of fee agreement.

Can executors be paid?

An executor is allowed to receive payment of a type via the will itself. A gift can be left in a will for the executor or trustees to express gratitude for the work they will do after the testator has died. A lawyer would normally charge a percentage of the value of the estate to do the probate or act as an executor and possibly an hourly fee. Lawyer's costs should be transparent and you can look online to find out what they should be. See the GOV.UK website for Solicitor's Guideline Hourly Rates.

Proprietary estoppel

Estoppel is a legal rule stopping a person from denying something they have previously said which someone else has relied on to their detriment. It may sound like intimidating legal jargon but it is an attempt by the legal system to make things fairer. So for example, if you have been promised your parents' hotel business with the expectation that you will work for the hotel for many years and contribute to it and then your parents die and it turns out they've left everything to a charity and you with nothing, you may have a claim. The idea is to provide some kind of recompense when children have contributed greatly to businesses because they have been told that they will inherit. With this expectation in mind, instead of seeking employment elsewhere they have worked long and hard to build up a business or improve a property only to find that they have been left little or nothing in the will.

Over the years there have been many court cases where an adult child has brought a claim against against their parent's estate for the above reasons. Many of these cases have involved farm properties where the child was encouraged to work on the farm for little or no wages on the basis that they would eventually inherit it but when the parent has died the child finds they have actually been left out. One case I find particularly interesting is that of Haberfield v Haberfield. A daughter worked for over fifty hours a week for thirty years on the family farm, having been told that she would be able to take it over when her father could no longer do it. The daughter said that her father had encouraged her to spend her time working on the farm and that when he was too elderly to run it himself, the understanding was that she would take over. Her mother denied this but the judge found in the daughter's favour. The daughter had been paid a lot less than someone would normally have been paid for this kind of work. The court decided that the daughter should receive compensation in a sum equivalent to the value of the part of the farm which had contained the dairy business. This had been promised to her and was therefore considered fair.

Property abroad

Many people now make more than one will. This has become quite common since we joined the EU and though we have left, many people still have a property abroad. This can complicate things if you're an executor because when your loved one dies you will have to get probate in the foreign country and sell the property. If you are a frequent visitor to the country you may want to look up some local solicitors in advance and see what services they offer. There are also many lawyers in the UK who specialise in the laws of other countries and speak the relevant language. There is currently a regulation called the 'European Succession Regulation' which, in very simple terms, means you can choose to have English law apply to your will in France, for example but this must be expressly stated in the will. This area of law is under revision and can become very complex if you have property in different countries or live in the UK but don't have British citizenship, so it is best to see a specialist lawyer about making a will when you have property abroad. You can find them by looking on the Law Society or The Notaries Society websites.

Marriage And Dementia

Dad is remarrying in his nineties. What if his wife to be is a fraudster? When it comes to marriage, both parties must have the mental capacity to understand what that commitment means. This has been confirmed by recent Court of Protection cases. You may know a vulnerable adult who seems happy to be getting married but underneath they may not really understand it or be able to consent to it. They could be subject to undue influence or coercion. A fraudster could simply be interested in inheriting money. Someone with dementia would be defined as a vulnerable adult and with that vulnerability comes issues surrounding their capacity to marry, the motivation of the person they are marrying and possible issues to do with who is going to look after who.

What do marriage officiants have to bear in mind? The government has published a Guide For The Clergy, which details what the clergy must check before a marriage takes place and A Guide For Authorised Persons which includes information about mental capacity and vulnerable adults, sham marriages and forced marriages. Both are published by GRO publishing and can be downloaded for free online.

If you are interested in case law on the subject of having the mental capacity to marry, a few recent Court of Protection cases are Mundell v Name 1 (2019), Southwark, (The London Borough of) v KA (Capacity to Marry) (2016) and BU, Re (2021).

Are you concerned that your elderly parent is getting involved with someone whose motives seem suspicious? There are orders that can be put in place called Forced Marriage Protection Orders. A forced marriage includes one that takes place using physical force, emotional pressure, threats or psychological abuse. The Forced Marriage Protection Order can help by stopping the perpetrator from contacting (directly or indirectly) the victim, from making wedding arrangements or being physically violent. This Order can be made in the Family Court and there is no court fee. You could get Legal Aid or bring the application yourself. You will find more information on the GOV.UK website.

It is important to remember that marriage automatically revokes a will. As previously mentioned, it is possible to make a will when you have dementia as long as the dementia is not too advanced and that decision must be made by a doctor. If a solicitor or will writer is not sure whether or not someone has capacity, they will ask a medical doctor to meet with the person and write a report about it, otherwise the will could be challenged. A will is invalid if a person makes or changes it without testamentary capacity. As an aside, it is possible to make a will in contemplation of marriage as long as the testator has capacity and this is something a will writer, lawyer or solicitor can do for you. However, the will must clearly state in writing that it is made in contemplation of marriage and will not be revoked by it and who the parties are.

<u>Moving in</u>

What if my loved one's partner moves in with them, what are my rights as a child of the house owner? This depends on whether or not the partner is contributing financially, for example paying rent, paying for an extension or paying for repairs etc. If they move in and they are not married to your parent, have not made any written agreement with them and they are making no financial contribution then they would have no more rights than any other guest in the home. There is a great deal of useful information on the internet in blogs written by lawyers covering subjects such as these where people are living together but not married. If your loved one then goes into a home and the partner stays in the house then it depends on who has a Lasting Power Of Attorney. If there is no power of attorney then again, an application to The Court Of Protection would unfortunately be needed.

If your relative dies and their partner remains in their house what happens? Assuming the partner is not in the will and the property is registered in the sole name of your loved one then the executors of the will would have a legal obligation to ask the partner to leave because the property would need to be passed down in accordance with the instructions in the will. If there is no will the property passes by the rules of intestacy in which case there will be 'administrators' rather than executors.

Deprivation Of Liberty Safeguards (DoLS)

Let's say your loved one has started to wander. One or two of the neighbours have started talking about this and saying that he or she seems to be crossing the road without really looking. They have accused you of not caring for your loved one properly. You ask the care agency to lock the house and leave the key in the key safe outside after they come round in the evening. Your loved one will therefore be unable to leave the house, thus keeping them safe from harm. Otherwise, you are afraid they may have an accident and may be hurt and you would never want to see them in pain. As well as this the neighbour's words are ringing in your head and you are afraid that any accident will be seen as your fault.

There are many awful things that could happen to an elderly person who is out alone, day or night. For example, being attacked, suffering from hypothermia or falling into water. You are feeling very scared about what might happen and it is on your mind all day. This is a totally unfair position for you to be in. You are damned if you do and damned if you don't. You are not a legal expert so how could you possibly know that not letting someone out of the house is against the law as it's an infringement of liberty and false imprisonment?

All you have done, out of the goodness of your heart, is try to protect your loved one and yourself. So what are you supposed to do? Only give them a key to the back door? That's not going to stop someone with dementia. A patient with dementia will climb fences, jump over hedges and go to the toilet in other people's gardens. If you ask them not to go out they may become aggressive. You will no doubt have already tried to discuss this with your loved one. If their dementia has progressed too far they may not really take this in but may be able to mask (pretend that they are just as they always were) very well. So your best option is to alert adult social services and let them know what is going on and to emphasise what a difficult position you are in. Tell them that without a DoLS you can't stop your loved one going out as it would be against the law to do so. You therefore need their advice as to what to do. Social services in England and Wales are hugely understaffed and overworked but you are really doing all you can by reporting your concerns. A social worker should come and do a mental capacity assessment (this can happen whilst you are present) and then you will be able to talk about your worries. The legal rules for situations where someone needs to be taken care of against their will are found in the Deprivation of Liberty Safeguards. These rules apply to situations where a person with dementia isn't able to consent to care. The Deprivation of Liberty Safeguards are an amendment to the Mental Capacity Act 2005 and they apply only in England and Wales. Don't necessarily rely on healthcare professionals to tell you this as they may not be up to date with all aspects of DoLS. As well as DoLS there is of course Article 5 of The Human Rights Act which is the right to liberty and security which prevents unlawful detention. Remember all this applies to you too. No one can force you to stay and look after an elderly relative. You too are free to leave.

If your relative is in a care home it will often be the care home manager who first mentions DoLS to you. If not, you may receive a phone call from a member of adult social services who will go through the process with you. They will explain what DoLS is and answer any questions you might have, they will enquire about your loved one and ask whether or not you agree that this is appropriate for them. They will explain that this is not so much about depriving a person of their freedom but about protecting them against going out alone, possibly having an accident or being taken advantage of in some way. The conversation will likely last about half an hour and after that they will confirm that a DoLS will be put in place. It is easier to do this when your loved one is in a care home. Most care homes will have a list of residents who are under a DoLS at the front desk and they will have someone on the front desk who monitors who goes in and out. Therefore you should not have to worry about this once your relative goes into the home and is under a DoLS. Having said that, it can take months for the DoLS application to go through and by the time you receive it from the local authority it may no longer be needed. Sadly, this was my experience. When it comes through you will receive an email from the county council's Deprivation of Liberty Team with attachments including: A Best Interest Assessor's Report, a Doctor's Report and a Standard Authorisation Granted document (which you will have to sign and send back). Additionally, there will be a letter explaining more about being a Relevant Person's Representative and a factsheet with further information. The DoLS usually lasts for twelve months after which it is reviewed.

A person with dementia who is in supported living can still be deprived of their liberty but this will usually only apply to people who need a great deal of care and support. The reason for this is that a person has to be constantly supervised in order for the DoLS to be effective. In this case the order should be authorised through the Court of Protection. They will carry out an independent mental assessment. You can find the form on the

GOV.UK website. It is Form COPDOL11 (Application to authorise a deprivation of liberty).

There is a new LPS (Liberty Protection Safeguards) coming in which is supposed to replace the Deprivation of Liberty Safeguards (DoLS). It was passed in May 2019 but is not yet in force. This will apply to people living in their own home or in supported living or who are part of the shared lives scheme (more on that later). This will mean that anyone who is going to be deprived of their liberty will be protected under the Liberty Protection Safeguards, without needing to go to court. Hopefully, this will speed things up and streamline the process because currently, in my opinion, the process is far too slow. It is regrettable that people such as busy social workers, care home staff and relatives are doing many hours of work preparing documentation which is never used because the vulnerable person dies before the DoLS is actually put in place. This seems to me to be an awful waste of time and resources as well as totally ineffective in terms of keeping the elderly safe.

Other Rights You May Have

Yes, you have rights! For example, you have the right to choose whether or not to be a carer, you have the right to provide some forms of care and not others because there are some elements of caring you may not feel comfortable with and you have the right to a Carer's Assessment. Here are some other carer's rights:

The Equality Act

If caring causes you to have a mental health issue or you already have one, or if it causes you to have a physical disability such as a back problem you may be protected under The Equality Act 2010.

The Equality Act says you have a disability if you have a 'mental or physical impairment' that has an adverse and long term effect on you and makes life difficult. For example, if you suffer from anxiety then it's going to be difficult for you to go to work every day; not only may you feel extremely afraid to go out of your house but your heart rate could be especially high and it may be very difficult to concentrate. In this case driving would be unwise. You may take medication such as propranolol or anti-depressants (the medication doesn't have to be specifically for a mental health issue). These medications may have side effects and again, your life could be substantially affected by these side effects. If you've suffered from anxiety for a year then that would be considered 'long term'. Even if your mental health issue gets better sometimes but it's likely to happen again then you should have certain protection against discrimination under the Act. Knowing you have this protection can be useful if you feel you have been treated unfairly by an employer who has perhaps put pressure on you to work too many hours, for example. You may also be protected under other laws including disability or sex discrimination laws.

Benefits

Turn2Us is a good website for checking eligibility for benefits. Unfortunately, benefit forms are becoming lengthier and lengthier which makes it harder for most people to apply for them. As usual, make sure you make a note of how much time you spend filling in the forms; it may be worth it if you manage to obtain some financial support.

When you finally get a dementia diagnosis for your loved one it is a good idea to get the doctor to complete a certificate for you. This certificate may help when you are applying for benefits such as attendance allowance, for example, or a council tax reduction.

And for you: Carer's Allowance (very little at approximately £80 per week) but be careful to check you are not earning a penny over the threshold! Otherwise the authorities could say that you have to pay back the carer's allowance. Yup, you know what I think about this. Perhaps authorities could make things a bit simpler for people who are already saving the country a huge amount of money and not penalise people who have made honest mistakes.

Additionally, you may be entitled to Carer's Credit. Although this benefit doesn't actually give you money in your pocket, it helps you to protect your pension and it may help when applying for other benefits. It is very useful if you are caring for someone but not paying National Insurance (NI) contributions because you are not going out to work. If you claim Carer's Credit you don't get a payment but you do get a NI contribution credit which goes on your pension record. You can look up your state pension summary by going to the National Insurance Page on the GOV.UK website.

At work

Going to work gets harder if you are a carer. There is much more work for you to do at home and this is combined with the worry that every time you leave the house your loved one could be in danger. Your employers should support you. They should not simply see it as an option. There are so many people who are carers now that it is in employers' interests to look after their employees in this regard. After all, this will make staff retention easier and save them money in the long run.

What rights do you have at work? You have the right to ask for flexible working hours and to take time off (although unpaid) during an emergency. Neither of these should affect your employment status. If you are starting a new job, find out what your workplace will be prepared to offer you and negotiate the best terms you can. Don't be afraid to talk openly about your caring responsibilities; you have a right to do so.

You may find there are special incentives for carers. Also, from April 2024, the new Carers Leave Act, means all unpaid carers will have the right to up to a week of unpaid leave to help with their caring responsibilities. This applies from the first day of your employment.

Carer's Week

A great way of raising awareness of how much work carers do is Carers' Week which is organised on an annual basis by Carers UK, a UK charity. Their goal, stated on the Charity Commission website is: 'To alleviate the conditions of life amongst people who are caring or who have cared for, elderly, sick, disabled or otherwise infirm persons' and to 'advance education concerning caring amongst carers and the public'. One really important aspect of their work is helping people to realise that they are carers in the first place. Many people don't think of themselves as carers and because of that they often don't even attempt to access the help and support they need. You can find out more about Carers' Week on their website. I really like the top ten activities they suggest for the week. These activities include sending hampers or care packages to carers and hosting an online quiz or coffee morning to enable new friends to be made.

Free vaccinations

If you give unpaid care to a loved one, you can ask your GP practice to put this on your patient record and you might get priority vaccinations like flu jabs or other benefits. The Carers UK website has a template letter you can use to send to your GP. You need to look after yourself in as many ways as you can when you are an unpaid carer.

Carer's Assessment

You also have a right to a Carer's Assessment if you are over eighteen and care for someone regularly and without payment. Often social services will initiate this once you have asked for a Care Needs Assessment for your relative but you can ask for it yourself. You can do this by contacting your local social services department. In Wales it is often called a Carer's Needs Assessment. A care assessor from the council will come and visit you (this could be done at the same time as your loved one's Needs Assessment). They will ask you questions about how you are managing, your health and how caring impacts your work and relationships. They may do a Careregiver's Strain Index questionnaire with you. This asks you questions such as, 'Is there anything the person you care for does that upsets you?' 'Is it a financial strain?' 'Is it a physical strain?' and so on. Do not be afraid to tell it how it is; they will have heard it all before. It is a good idea to ask specifically about respite in advance so that you can get a break.

What Is An Attorney And Do I Have To Be One?

Lasting Powers of Attorney are documents that enable someone or more than one person to act on another's behalf. They were created by the Mental Capacity Act 2005. You do not have to be one if you don't want to be. As an attorney for your elderly parent you will do hours of work. It tends to be sold to you as a power that gives you rights. In fact it is another unpaid job. It is an onerous job; not only in the preparation of the documents themselves; The Lasting Power of Attorney For Finance and The Lasting Power of Attorney for Health and Welfare, but in the carrying out of those duties. Lasting powers of attorney can be made online on the government website and you can also find out if someone already has an LPA by looking on the same site.

What does the job involve? Being an attorney for finance involves managing the donor's bank accounts, buying food and clothes for the donor, dealing with insurance companies, energy providers, care agencies and care homes, keeping accounts and all receipts, (even pestering shop assistants when they run out of receipt roll to give you a hand written one!), making sure the donor's money is protected, managing savings, premium bonds, investment portfolios, taxes, bills, houses, businesses and state benefits, charities, intellectual property etc (it's not an exhaustive list). You will need time and organisational skill to do this job and it is preferable if you are younger than the donor and relatively healthy. If your loved one also has a business it may be a good idea to have a Lasting Power of Attorney for Business too as a colleague may not wish to make decisions on their behalf or may not be able to; it depends on what kind of business it is and how the decisions are made. Bills and salaries will need to be paid and someone will have to have overall responsibility.

There are many advantages to LPAs; being able to deal with property and bank accounts, not having to apply for a deputyship order, being able to deal with care homes and have your loved one admitted to a care home. Most care homes now require both LPAs to admit a resident. The reason for this is that if a difficult situation arises, such as a need to make quick decisions about a resident's care then the home manager can look to the attorney for health and welfare to provide an answer. The need for an attorney for finance is obvious since the care home will be accepting payments from the power of attorney account into their own business bank account.

Your loved one can put specific clauses in the Lasting Power of Attorney according to their wishes and this often makes things much clearer and saves any guesswork on your part. For example, in a finance and property LPA they could write, in the guidance section: 'I prefer to invest in ethical funds'. If the donor wishes to pay an amount to the attorney/s they could also write something like, *'Each attorney must be paid £2,000 per year'*. Obviously, the fees will come out of the donor's funds. If the donor doesn't record their wishes regarding payment here then non-professional attorneys can only get paid back expenses and to recover these they will need to keep receipts. Expenses include things like postage, travel and accountancy. In the Health and Welfare LPA you can specify on the preferences and instructions page such things as the medical treatment you would prefer, who you want to have contact with (this could be useful if you fall out with a particular family member) and even what kind of social activities you want to do (if you don't fancy knitting or poetry you shouldn't be made to write a poem about Fair Isle!). If the donor wishes to continue to pay any charities or expenses, even when they are not living in the property but are living in a care home, they should state this in the LPA.

When you take over your loved one's bills, don't be afraid to challenge them. You may need to send utility companies copies of the LPAs by email but they are usually pretty quick in dealing with this. You can then email them or, through their portals, update and possibly reduce the bills. It's a good idea to take photos (time and date stamped on your phone) of meter readings and so on and the Citizens Advice Bureau have a dedicated team who deal with issues with energy providers. It's always a good idea to log your case with the CAB at the same time as you are writing to the energy provider and let them know you have done this.

What happens when your loved one can no longer manage their money? If you find they have stashed hundreds of pounds under the mattress and are constantly going to the bank and taking out large sums of cash you can, with an LPA for Finance and Property, bring up the issue with the bank. They can reduce the limit on withdrawals, turn off contactless payments, or set up alerts for you. You could also set up another account under your LPA, keep a lower amount of money in it and give your loved one a card for that. These are all just ideas but you might find some of them helpful.

What about health and welfare? Being an attorney for health and welfare involves making decisions about day to day care, medicines, life sustaining treatment such as DNRs (do not resuscitate orders; more on them later) and pain relief when the person is dying. You can also ask your relative's doctor to give you access to their medical records. In order to do this, if you don't have an LPA for Health and Welfare, you would have to fill in a form given to you by the doctor and your loved one will have to sign it to give you permission to access their records. They will have to have the mental capacity to sign this at the time that they do it.

When can I step in as an attorney? In both types of LPA you can take over when the donor doesn't have capacity. So let's say someone had mental capacity but then had an accident and went into a coma then the LPAs could be used. If that person then came out of their coma and regained mental capacity the attorneys could stand down until such time as the power of attorney was needed again. There are helpful guides to filling in the Lasting Power of Attorney on the GOV.UK website. Once your elderly relative loses capacity you will have to produce the registered LPAs quite often and it's a good idea to have them scanned so you can email them to the relevant organisations and companies when necessary.

LPA jargon

What does 'joint and several' mean when talking about how attorneys can make decisions? (This will appear in Section 3 of the LPA form which the donor must fill in). What it means is that you can make some decisions together with the other attorneys and some separately. To make decisions 'jointly' means you have to make every decision together unanimously which could be very time consuming. Imagine if your brother or sister lives in New Zealand and you live in England. Every time a decision has to be made, be it big or small, you are going to have to call or email them and wait for a response. If you are 'joint and several' attorneys then it means one of you can go ahead and buy clothes for your loved one, or contact the doctor to do a pain medication review, straight away. If a dispute arises between you and the other attorney/s and it's about something serious then, if you couldn't solve it by mediation you would have to go to court to sort it out. Additionally if something happens to one attorney the other can always take over if needed as long as the donor chooses the 'joint and several' option.

What happens if you do something wrong?

Most people who are caring for someone with dementia are not doing anything wrong and even if they are technically doing something wrong, it is unlikely they are aware of it. It is much more likely that they are so exhausted in their caring role that they have no further mental energy to investigate every nuance of the power of attorney role or the law. They are also unlikely to have the money to go and see a lawyer who would be able to examine their particular situation in detail.

But in order to protect yourself, if you stick to the basic principle that you can't spend money on yourself that is the donor's money, unless it is explicitly stated in the Power of Attorney, you shouldn't go far wrong. Having it stated in the Power of Attorney saves any worry for you. You can look at the guidance on the Office of the Public Guardian website about giving gifts or contact them to check if they consider that you are doing the right thing. If you do contact the Office of the Public Guardian, keep any copies of correspondence and make notes of any calls and the date and time you made them. You can do this if you are in any way unsure of what you are buying and spending money on. Always keep receipts for everything you buy in a separate folder and originals or electronic copies of any bills or anything that comes out by direct debit.

The examples I was able to find on the internet regarding gifts did not cover enough potential scenarios in my opinion. Unfortunately, the Mental Capacity Act 2005 doesn't define what is a 'reasonable' or 'unreasonable' gift and the Office of the Public Guardian doesn't give exact figures. You are expected to decide how much is reasonable (in my opinion, more detailed guidance is needed for unpaid carers). You are allowed to give money to family and friends in small amounts. So for example, if your loved one would normally have bought their grandchildren gifts for Christmas worth £30 each then it is reasonable to think that they would have approved of you doing this on their behalf. Obviously, you also have to take into account how much money there is left in their account. Bear in mind that what the will says is a separate issue so you can't use the donor's money in the way their will says while they are still alive. The Lasting Power of Attorney dies with the donor and the will only takes effect after death.

If the donor, before losing capacity, had financially provided for a dependent or relative, then it is not unreasonable to conclude that they would want this to continue. Once again, it's a good idea to plan in advance if you can and look at what they are likely to be able to afford over the coming years taking into account the huge cost of care fees. If in doubt, to protect yourself against those who may accuse you of fraud, apply to the Court of Protection to make the decision as to whether you can continue to make payments to someone who is dependent on the donor. A gift from the donor's account could include making a loan from the donor's funds. To use the LPA for that you will need to apply to the Court of Protection. Once you have applied, the Court of Protection will either approve or refuse your request.

When it comes to selling a house you will need to talk to a solicitor though you can do this with an LPA as long as there are no restrictions in it. Sadly, property fraud is becoming so prevalent that conveyancers are having to take every precaution they legally can in order to satisfy their insurers so don't be offended if they ask you lots of questions, it's nothing personal. After all, think how you would feel if a conveyancer sold your parent's house to a buyer only to find out that the seller was not your parent or their attorney but someone pretending to be them while they were abroad or in hospital.

Should anyone challenge your spending they should make sure they know what they are talking about and have material evidence to prove that you have spent money contrary to the best interests of the donor. If anyone, including friends or relatives, challenge your spending your counter argument will be that you have cared for your relative for x number of years and that the current rate of pay for a live in carer is £x amount which usually adds up to hundreds of thousands of pounds over the period of time you have been doing it. Additionally, you have probably looked after the house, done all the repairs, worked unpaid as an attorney, registered an LPA which would probably cost around £900 for two if you were to have it done by a solicitor, done hours of work filling in forms etc. If you add up all this unpaid work you will soon have a good counter argument. Your time is important and it should never be underestimated.

Can I walk away?

Yes you can! You can renounce your attorneyship and in fact all your caring responsibilities and go and live in another country if you want to. I remember pointing this out to a social worker once. He suddenly went quiet and after a long pause, reluctantly agreed with me. Once you have renounced your attorneyship you can't reapply though; it's not something you can put down and pick up on a whim.

Why would you want to renounce the attorneyship? Life happens! Things change! Finances can become more complex as time goes on, or an attorney might become ill or find that they have many other responsibilities they did not expect. Increasingly, as people are living into their nineties, their children are in their seventies by the time they become attorneys. In this case it may be wise to let someone younger take on the role.

In order to stop being an attorney before the donor dies (this is called 'disclaiming' an attorneyship) you have to fill in an OPG (Office of the Public Guardian) form LPA005. This can be downloaded from their website. However, you should talk to a qualified lawyer initially or get some good advice because you don't want to leave the donor without any attorneys as this would invalidate the LPA. They will be able to tell you how to retire as an attorney without causing any issues for yourself or the donor. Perhaps a replacement attorney can take over.

When the donor wants to replace an attorney

For one reason or another a donor may want to remove or replace an attorney and this can be done as long as they still have capacity. Because relationships and personal situations change over time, it's a really good idea to update your healthcare and financial powers of attorney every few years. You can revoke an LPA by going on the GOV.UK website. What you do is notify all the attorneys and tell them about the revocation, telling them not to use their powers. You complete the revocation forms and a Deed of Revocation. You can then submit a new LPA. If you want to appoint new attorneys then you send the Office of the Public Guardian the replacement LPA which names your new attorneys. Obviously it's a good idea for your loved one to quickly make a new LPA to avoid a situation where they don't have one but then lose capacity.

In order to remove an attorney under an Enduring Power of Attorney (EPA) you would have to revoke the EPA. Enduring Powers of Attorney aren't made any more though the ones that were created before LPAs came in are still valid. So in this case the donor would revoke the EPA and then make two new LPAs instead. This can be done as long as the donor still has mental capacity.

If your loved one doesn't have an LPA and they have lost mental capacity then a family member may need to apply to the Court of Protection to become a deputy. A deputy has similar powers to an attorney and can manage the individual's finances. Try if you possibly can to avoid this situation. The process of appointing a deputy is longer, more complicated and more expensive than registering an LPA. You will have to have your accounting monitored regularly. The cost is about £1,000 if it includes a hearing and then there is an annual supervision fee, so it's quite an intrusive and expensive process.

Advance Directives/Advance Decisions/Living Wills

Why does the same thing have three names? As if one weren't enough! An Advance Directive (sometimes known as an Advance Decision or a Living Will) tells others what medical treatment you would like to receive if you are unable to communicate those wishes in the future. For example, how you would want to be made comfortable if you were suffering from a terminal illness. As long as the Advance Directive is properly drawn up it is legally binding on medical professionals. However, there are restrictions. You can't use an Advance Directive to refuse basic care such as being kept comfortable and pain free. This is because sudden withdrawal of pain medication could be unsafe and doctors, nurses and carers could be put in impossible and unfair situations. You can refuse life-sustaining treatment (life sustaining treatment is medical intervention to prolong life) in an Advance Directive, but if you want to do this make sure you use the correct wording or seek professional advice as there are some technical considerations.

The main advantage of an Advance Directive is that it's effective as soon as it's made and does not need to be registered before it can be used. This is a big plus particularly if a person has a terminal illness or suddenly goes downhill. They are also good if you have personal beliefs about medical treatment. Health workers are not psychic and have hundreds of patients to look after so it helps if the Advance Directive is in your loved one's file at the care home. It is hard enough to know what a patient wants, especially if they have dementia and are finding it hard to communicate. If they have been able to make an Advance Directive you will not have to race around trying to find out from other relatives what they wanted at what will be a very stressful time.

What's an Advance Statement?

An Advance Statement, unlike an Advance Directive, is not legally binding, but anyone who's making decisions about your care must take account of it. Sometimes it's included in an Advance Directive in a special section. An Advance Statement can include your religious or spiritual beliefs, how you don't want to live, how you like to do things; for example, do you prefer to have a bath or a shower? Do you like to sleep with the lights on? Do you have any pets and if you became ill who would look after them? You can talk to relatives and friends about your statement and make them aware of where you have kept it so that it is easily accessible should you have to go into care.

Having an Advance Statement will help care home staff to understand you and get to know you quickly. It will avoid any potential misunderstandings. I know of one person who is afraid of dogs and another who loves them. Since dogs often accompany their owners to care homes it is helpful for the care home staff to know in which direction to steer them!

How Advance Directives and LPAs are different

In a Health and Welfare LPA you are appointing other people: 'attorneys', to make decisions for you when you lose capacity. You are providing them with some instructions on how they can do this on your behalf. In an Advance Directive on the other hand, you are telling people what kinds of treatment you do and don't want in the future; there's no attorney. So both documents protect your interests but in different ways. You can have an

Advance Directive and a Health and Welfare LPA at the same time but just be careful they don't conflict because otherwise if you make an Advance Directive first and then your LPA the LPA will override the Advance Directive and vice versa. Both an Advance Directive and a Lasting Power of Attorney come to an end when a person dies. The Advance Directive can give your attorney extra insight into the kind of care you want.

Deputies

If someone seems to have no one looking after them you can search the government's website under the section headed: Searching our registers of attorneys, deputies and guardians (Form OPG 100). The search is free.

In the case that someone is vulnerable and starting to suffer from dementia then you can apply to become a deputy for them if they have no one else. You can apply to be a deputy for finance and/or health and welfare. However, you will have to fill in forms and this is quite complex. There are instructions on the website but it is an expensive application and costs around £400 to make. You will have to send a deputy report to the Office of the Public Guardian every year justifying your decisions and you may also have to set up a bond with a security bond provider (if you are a finance deputy). A representative from the Court of Protection may visit you to make sure you are fulfilling your duties. You will also have to pay an annual supervision fee and possibly an assessment fee. So this is not an easy job and is not to be taken lightly. You are only allowed to make the decisions the court has ordered you can make and you should have a good knowledge of the Mental Capacity Act 2005. If there's no one else to be a deputy then a professional deputy needs to be appointed. This should be a qualified and experienced lawyer. As a professional they will be entitled to be paid as they will have to spend hours reviewing all decisions made, among other things. Costs could be more than £10,000 a year plus VAT.

Decision makers

When there is no Power of Attorney, certain people may become decision-makers under the Mental Capacity Act 2005. The decision-makers could be carers, doctors, nurses, social workers or police for example. They must, of course, make decisions in the person's best interests and there is guidance given by the OPG and NICE (The National Institute For Health And Care Excellence) as to what this entails.

Appointees

Sometimes it is possible to become an 'appointee' for someone who loses mental capacity if they don't have an LPA. As long as the vulnerable person only has pensions and benefits you could apply to the Department for Work and Pensions (DWP) to become their appointee. You would then be able to manage that person's benefits and state pension. In this case, a Deputyship Order could be avoided.

Disadvantages of a Power of Attorney

Being an attorney has its downsides. Not only is it a huge amount of work but anyone; a carer, a neighbour, a friend, colleague or a professional can report an attorney to the Office of The Public Guardian for misuse of the donor's funds. They can do this via the website of the Office of the Public Guardian. Having said this, they must have some evidence of the accusation and it is a long and detailed form to fill in. To raise a concern about an attorney, you have to use form OPG130 or write directly to the Office of the Public Guardian. A person cannot simply raise a concern because they see that an attorney has been on holiday or bought a new car. That a carer should have to worry about being reported when they desperately need a holiday is a sad state of affairs. I think there should be much more clarity around these issues.

If someone reports you to the Office of the Public Guardian there are lawyers who can help. Go to the internet and type in: 'False accusations of LPA abuse' and you should be able to find specialist lawyers in your area. The Citizens Advice Bureau are also extremely helpful.

The reality is that most attorneys don't do anything wrong deliberately, they are just trying to navigate an extremely complex situation at an extremely stressful time. Even most lawyers don't know the ins and outs of the law of attorneyship. It is a very specialised area. If you are investigated by the Office of the Public Guardian it may not result in any action being taken against you at all, it may be that you are simply given guidance on how to carry on with your role. Just because an investigation has been carried out it doesn't mean any fraud has taken place or anyone has done anything wrong; it is just a safeguard. Also, the Office of the Public Guardian must take into account the fact that people have the human right to privacy and family life.

Lasting Power of Attorney fraud is a real worry. Lawyers have warned that a fraudster could submit a 'complete work of fiction' to the government body overseeing the scheme, with falsified names and addresses and be handed the legal document entitling them to take over the affairs of the victim. Victim's empty homes have been targeted by fraudsters who obtained an LPA without any proper checks. The fraudsters briefly visited the woman's flat to drill out the locks and then tried to sell it using the document. So it pays to keep checks on your loved one's property whether they are living in it or not.

Independent Mental Capacity Advocates

If the person has no attorney, no deputy and no close friends or family they may be appointed an Independent Mental Capacity Advocate (IMCA). Again, these were introduced by the Mental Capacity Act 2005. As with other health professionals, all IMCA's must have enhanced DBS checks and IMCA training with recognised bodies. They can help with medical treatment or living accommodation or when someone who lacks capacity is in a situation where they need to be protected (in cases of alleged abuse). They can also visit a vulnerable person wherever they are living and can help them to communicate with other people who look after them. If the vulnerable person wishes to complain about their care the IMCA can help with this too. There are websites such as SWAN (South West Advocacy Network) which are quite accessible and easy to read. The Department of Health also has an IMCA website with the details of all IMCA providers.

Funding, The Local Authority And The NHS

You are not legally liable to pay for your elderly parent's care. There are no filial responsibility laws in England and Wales. In a care home or nursing home, people with assets of more than £24,000, and that may include the value of any property they own, may have to pay for the cost of their care (at time of writing). Hopefully this will change in the future because caring for an elderly relative can be financially disastrous. You are trying to juggle work, caring for others and caring for them. You can't live on carer's allowance so you have to work. Some people give up work because understandably they can't do two or three jobs at the same time. In the end they may have to eat up savings, cash in their pensions or borrow money and this may result in getting into debt. It's yet another stress when you least need it.

How to get a dementia diagnosis

Getting a diagnosis is a good starting point. It is worrying when you start to notice that your elderly relative is forgetting things on a regular basis. They may be asking the same questions again and again or finding it hard to use a cash machine. You may notice that they have started writing notes to themselves with names, appointments or instructions on how to do simple things. The collection of papers increases until one day you realise you can't see the furniture under them. So how do you get a diagnosis from a doctor when your loved one doesn't want to go and refuses to believe there is anything wrong with them? You could suggest that you and your loved one go to the doctor for a check up. You could call the surgery in advance and ask if they can include a dementia assessment. They will usually do this in a sensitive way, framing it as a general check up. There isn't one single test for dementia at the moment. Dementia testing can be done at the GP practice or at a memory clinic. The tests are called 'cognitive assessments' and your loved one may also be invited to have scans, such as CT scans or MRI scans on another day to ensure the diagnosis is correct. The GP will need to look at your relative's medical history to see if there are any contributing factors to their memory loss. They may also do blood tests as some other conditions can cause mental confusion or dementia-like symptoms, such as liver and kidney problems. You can attend if you want to and it may help as you will be able to describe any problems you've noticed. There are several different tests that the GP can use. The General Practitioner Assessment of Cognition (GPCOG) is one such test. You can find this online under GPCOG. It's a popular option because it's quick and can be used in most settings. The GP might ask you some questions too, such as, how has your loved one changed in the last five years? Are they able to manage public transport? And so on.

How to get funding – formophobia!

The first step in obtaining funding is getting what is called a 'Care Needs Assessment'. This is free and anyone can ask for one. In order to get a Care Needs Assessment you can contact social services and ask. Or you can do it online on the GOV.UK website. Yet more formophobia! But unfortunately, this is the only way to get the ball rolling and engage social services. A needs assessment can take place online, by phone or face to face. Usually a social worker will come round to the house and have a chat. This will include discussing how easily they can do everyday activities such as move around, cook or shower. If the social worker thinks grab rails or a bath seat may be beneficial then a home assessment can take place. You can talk to your loved one about their needs before the assessment so that you are both prepared. If social services say nothing is needed and you disagree you have a right to complain. You can complain to your local council (usually done on their website) or if you're not happy with their response you can complain to the local government and social care ombudsman. They have a website which gives you a step-by-step guide to making a complaint.

Financial Assessment

If the care needs assessment identifies your loved one needs help, they will then have a Financial Assessment (means test) to see if the council will pay towards their care. This will be arranged for you but you may have to wait quite a while! I think I waited at least three months for my initial phone call. Social services will eventually phone you and/or the care home to get some initial information. After a few more weeks you will get another call which goes into a bit more depth (this is from an assessor who will then pass on your information to the adult social worker in your area). They will then call you and arrange to meet up with you both either at the care home or your own home. Usually they will sit down with you and ask a few simple questions such as how long has your loved one been in the home? Where did they last live? What are their interests? This is for the purpose of finding out a bit about them and also ascertaining their current level of cognition. If your relative is already a resident in a care home the social worker will want to know if you are both happy with the level and type of care being given and if the care home is able to provide the necessary facilities. The reason for this is that some care homes don't have the capacity to look after residents who have certain needs or they may not have staff with the appropriate training for dementia. In this case you can look for a home that is more suitable. You and the social worker may then go and have a chat independently and you will need to produce the Lasting Powers of Attorney for Health and Finance (you can send them to the social worker by email if you like). Assessments usually last at least an hour.

Sometimes, in the course of these appointments, a social worker or other professional may ask if they can speak with your loved one alone. Don't be offended by this, it is standard practice and nothing personal at all. It actually protects you against being accused of undue influence etc. So think of it as a form of self protection.

After the meeting with the social worker you will be asked to sign some documents to allow the local authority to access your loved one's medical records and confirm that you have authority such as an LPA. You also need to sign a statement that says your relative's income can be used towards their care home fees. The social worker will then chat to the home manager and you can ask any questions you have such as when the outcome will be known or when the care home will receive the first payment.

Incidentally, you can stay living at home when your loved one moves into a care home and in fact it may be a good idea as you will be able to look after the property (properties fall into disrepair very quickly when no one is living in them). Make sure to check the home and contents insurance and let the insurers know too.

The request for local authority funding will be either discretionary or mandatory. It will be mandatory if you are over sixty, under eighteen or disabled (more on that in a minute). Finally, the social worker will produce a report, which they will share with you. This will outline your loved one's needs and what care is recommended. Once you have checked the details it will be passed to the social worker's manager for sign off and then sent to the local authority for a decision. This may take months; in my case it took eight.

What if I am living in the property?

You may be living in the same property as your elderly relative. This can happen for many reasons, such as, you have been caring for them for years, they have asked you not to leave them alone or you have never been able to get on the property ladder due to lack of money or disability. If this is the case, and the house is in your loved one's name, you may be eligible for what is called a 'relative's property disregard'. This means when you apply for local authority funding they cannot include the value of the property in the calculation. The child, partner or relative must have lived in the property as their main or only home since before the resident entered the care home. You can find more details on GOV.UK under Relative's Property Disregard which will also give you a definition of what is considered a relative. This includes a parent in law, step-parent, or sibling. Make sure you apply at least ten months in advance of the money running out. I was never able to find anyone who could give me a time estimate for how long it would take to get a decision on funding. There are time estimates given on government websites for other services and it would have been really helpful to have had this in regard to a funding decision.

If you are over the age of sixty and are living in the same house as your relative you should automatically get the property disregard. Effectively, this means that the local authority can't touch the house you are living in. If you are under sixty and are living in the property, you may still be eligible for a property disregard if you are claiming a disability benefit. In this way, you will get funding for your loved one to stay in a care or nursing home, rather than having a 'charge' on the house in the form of a deferred payment agreement (see below). In my opinion this is very unfair because many people fall just outside the criteria for being able to apply for benefits and the government are making it harder and harder to get them. However, if you are already claiming a disability benefit this may help you with local authority care funding.

You can also request a discretionary property disregard if you have acted as your relative's carer over a period of years and you have lived in their property. You would need to give the local authority details of the caring role you have played including how many hours per week you have worked as a carer. Let's face it; most carers work for their loved one all week, twenty four seven, and they care physically and psychologically. I had to write what amounted to a short novel about the caring I had done for my mother and how long I had done this for. I also had to write in detail about my anxiety and depression. I was told the discretionary property disregard panel would only consider my case if I had made 'considerable savings to the public purse!'. As mentioned above I consider that unpaid carers already save the public purse £13.9 billion every year but I suppose there are people out there who pretend to be carers when they aren't so perhaps that is why we have to jump through so many hoops. If the panel agree with the case you put forward then the property will be disregarded whilst you continue to live there. If neither of the above apply, then the local authority could offer you a deferred payment agreement.

What is a Deferred Payment Agreement?

This is an arrangement whereby the local council will put a charge on an owner's house that allows them to use the equity in the house for the care home costs. This means that the property will not have to be sold in your relative's lifetime. A charge is a legal interest in a property which is created to secure debt, a bit like a mortgage. This will appear on the title deeds showing that the local council have a right to get back the money loaned from the net proceeds of sale of the property. This is standard practice when you are taking out a loan on a property because obviously the lender will want to make sure they are going to get their money back eventually. You can view the title deeds (it costs about £7) on the Land Registry website and you will be able to see that they have entered a charge on the property as it will appear under the section named, 'charges'. If you qualify for a deferred payment agreement, the council will pay the care home bills and you don't have to pay them back until your loved one has died. The money to pay back the council will be repaid when the property is sold. Of course you could also get a private loan but be very careful about repayment charges and interest and get good financial advice before you consider this option.

Equity release

Equity release should be mentioned here but the interest rates can be high so be aware of this. Most people know that it's a way of using the equity in a property to obtain cash to clear debts or pay for care. But be careful with this as it is one of the most expensive options and can be a burden for life. It is best to go and see an independent financial advisor if you are considering this option. The two common types of equity release products in the UK are lifetime mortgages and home reversion plans. With a lifetime mortgage you repay the money you've borrowed once you sell the property. Whereas with a home reversion plan you sell part or all of your property to a home reversion provider. You get a lump sum or a regular income but can stay living in the property. As with the lifetime mortgage, when the property is sold the provider will get their money back from the proceeds of sale. Any interest by any party in a property is recorded on the Land Registry title deeds. You may find that equity release companies do not like other lenders having charges registered against the property. They will want to be the only ones to have a charge. Therefore, part of the process of getting equity release, if there are already other charges on the property, will be paying back the previous charges and clearing them from the Land Registry register.

What if they don't help me?
If you don't agree with the council's decision about care home funding you have the right to challenge it. You can do this if they refuse to pay for care, if you're unhappy with the service you've received or if you don't think they're offering enough towards care costs.

The process is as follows: First of all you complain directly to your local council. All councils should have a complaints procedure on their websites so you can fill in an online form or phone them. If you're still not happy with the way the council handles your complaint, you can take it to the Local Government and Social Care Ombudsman. An ombudsman should be independent and look thoroughly into your complaint. They will investigate to find out whether or not you have suffered loss, harm or distress as a result of the service provider's failings. They can investigate and can take action as long as you aren't currently taking legal action of your own against the authority. If you live in Wales you can contact the Public Service Ombudsman (PSO) for Wales. They can deal with complaints about most public bodies such as councils and housing associations and the website has a complaints form you can fill in. (Their telephone number is: 0300 790 0203 and their website is: www.ombudsman.wales).

Immediate Needs Annuity

What is an Immediate Needs Annuity? Anyone over the age of sixty can apply for an Immediate Needs Care Annuity (also called a Care Fee Plan) if they have to be cared for in a residential setting or at home and they are self-funding. An Immediate Needs Annuity is similar to an ordinary annuity except the income you receive goes towards your care costs. So it's an insurance policy where you can pay a lump sum to the insurance company and you get a regular income back which you can use to pay care costs. One of the advantages is that this doesn't count as income, so you don't pay income tax on it. How it works is that you pay a lump sum into the annuity and the annuity pays the care provider. The issue with this is you will need to agree how much the upfront payment will be and it could be quite a large amount; we're talking thousands of pounds, so it may be as much as the value of a property; not something everyone can afford to do.

But what happens if your loved one dies within a few months of setting this up? Does the estate get the money back? Well, they can include a clause in the contract which is called a 'capital protection clause' which says that the beneficiaries will receive part of the lump sum if the owner of the annuity dies early. However, the original lump sum might have to be quite high and you might get back less money than you originally paid in. There should be a cooling off period of thirty days. Additionally, the annuity payments may affect your eligibility for certain benefits. You can find Immediate Needs Annuity calculators online, though most ask for an email address in order to send you a quote. Each annuity will be different as it is based on the applicant's medical records, age and so on. Of course, m*edical records have to be provided too. After a few weeks they should send you a quote.* Be careful though, if you become eligible for another type of funding you might not be able to cancel your Immediate Needs Annuity and if you do get some of it back, it could be subject to income tax at that point.

You can also get what is called a Deferred Needs Care Annuity. This can be used when you think you might need to pay care costs in the future. It works in the same way as an Immediate Needs Annuity except that the income is, obviously, paid at some time in the future when you need care.

Renting
Renting a room, house or flat is another option to help pay care home fees. This is something you can do if you and another attorney have an LPA for property and finance. Doing this could be difficult if your loved one has been a hoarder. There may be years and years of paperwork or belongings that have been stored and you will need to deal with this in order to make room for a tenant and/or refurbish the property or room. Again, you

should consider some kind of tenancy agreement and get the necessary insurance.

Health insurance

Some insurance companies are beginning to offer products to help with the costs of dementia care in later life. This can be added on to serious illness cover and may be a way of paying for some of the costs of care in later life. The payment will go directly to the policy holder in the event they are diagnosed with dementia. These can be found online.

Benevolent funds

Benevolent funds are types of charities which were originally set up to help people who had worked in a certain profession and fallen on hard times. We are now living in a time of extreme financial hardship for all but a lucky few and these benevolent funds are more needed than ever before. They can help with respite breaks and funeral costs as well as counselling and mental health support. The Association of Charitable Organisations can help you get information about these benevolent societies and charities. Alternatively, a full list of benevolent funds and charities can be found on the Carer's Trust Website. Turn2US is also a good website for finding out about charities, funds and grants and Christians Against Poverty may also be able to help.

Credit unions may be able to offer you more flexible accounts than a bank due to their focus on customer service rather than profit. They are owned by their members, rather than by shareholders or investors and so may be better for those who can't easily access mainstream financial products. It's worth shopping around to find the best deals though as it really depends on your own circumstances and you might get cheaper deals with other financial institutions.

What about ethical banking? This is a bank that follows a set of principles in order to try and improve society or the environment. So it might, for example, give loans to charities or it may refuse to invest in weapons or tobacco. You may prefer to use this kind of bank for altruistic reasons.

NHS Continuing Healthcare Funding

There are thousands of people caring for loved ones in their homes, often under agonising levels of stress. Others spend their life savings and sell their homes to pay care home fees. Many of these people should have got NHS Continuing Healthcare Funding. This is completely separate from local authority funding and is not means-tested. I found it very difficult to get any information about this from professionals when I was looking after mum; it seems it is a well-kept secret! It is a complex application process and I was told that it is very rare that someone gets this funding when they are already in a care home, as opposed to a nursing home. It is a person's day-to-day healthcare needs that matter, rather than their diagnosis. However, I think it's worth trying to get this; even if the funding the NHS provides is not enough to pay the full costs of care, you may be able to get a certain percentage of it paid. It may also be worth appealing for retrospective funding if you don't get it straight away, even after your loved one has passed away. If they have recently been discharged from hospital they may be entitled to six weeks of free care in a care home so don't give up!

What does NHS Continuing Healthcare Funding cover? It can cover all care fees for those who need full-time care due to a serious health condition so you may qualify for NHS Continuing Healthcare Funding if you have a 'primary health need'. This means that the majority of care given must involve managing health needs, rather than social or personal care needs. Certain criteria have to be met. For example, there has to be a need for prescriptions, injections and medical equipment for the patient to survive.

The full criteria are in the National Framework for NHS Continuing Healthcare and NHS-Funded Nursing Care (2018). So for example, if your loved one has dementia and also has a serious physical disability such as partial paralysis, they could apply for this type of funding. It covers the full cost of your care (in your own home or a nursing home), including healthcare, personal care and care home fees. It is not about where you live or whether or not you have a house. If you are providing your loved one with care at home, Continuing Healthcare Funding should cover all nursing care and personal care such as bathing and dressing. It may also cover household expenses related to care needs such as accessible vehicle costs, laundry services and incontinence pads.

If you've spoken to people in health and social care about paying care home fees and they've been vague or unhelpful it may be because they know little about the legal context in which they work. This is not their fault. The legal system of the NHS is not exactly streamlined, being a complex combination of case law, common law and statute! So don't expect them to necessarily give you correct information about care fees. It is best to do your own research. Say your loved one is in hospital after a stroke and after many weeks you meet the discharge coordinator who says they have to go home now and no more can be done for them in hospital. It's a good thing they own their home, they say, they will be able to use this to fund their own care. But this is not strictly true; the fact is you don't necessarily have to sell the house to pay for care. As soon as your loved one goes into a care home or nursing home get them assessed for Continuing Healthcare Funding. Only if Local Authority Funding and NHS Continuing Healthcare Funding has been applied for and refused can your relative be asked to self -fund.

The first thing that should happen in every case is an assessment of health and care needs, it shouldn't matter how much money someone has. There should be an assessment for NHS Continuing Healthcare Funding at the very beginning. How do I get this? You ask. Go to a GP, social worker or nurse and get them to do an evaluation to find out if your loved one is eligible. You may find email contact details for your local ICB (Integrated Care Board) team on their website. If your loved one's health is getting worse quickly you should ask to get a fast-track assessment. You can start by going to their GP. When I phoned up a hospice and a GP no one knew anything about NHS Continuing Healthcare Funding; the hospice told me to go back to the GP and the GP told me to go to PALS (the Patient Liaison Service at the local hospital). You will need to be insistent. I have to admit I gave up at the time because of the levels of stress I was under but it shouldn't be that way. People should be given much more assistance with this in the places they go to when they are in crisis.

One way to get a fast-track funding assessment is to go to the GOV.UK website and print out the NHS Continuing Healthcare Funding fast-track pathway tool form. You could then take that to the GP and ask them to either fill in the form themselves or get an appropriate healthcare worker to do it. Obviously, you want your loved one to get the best care possible if they are at the end of life stage and any funding you can get is going to help them. The GP should send the completed form to the local ICB.

If you are told your loved one is not eligible for funding you can ask your ICB to reconsider. Once that has happened if you still disagree with the decision or they way they handled the matter, you can ask for a review by NHS England. After this, if the original decision is still upheld you have the right to make a complaint to the Parliamentary and Health Service Ombudsman. Anyone has a right to complain about the service they receive from the NHS or the local authority and that is as it should be. The complaints procedures are all available from the above organisation's websites. Be sure to appeal any Continuing Healthcare Funding decision you disagree with. If you have the time and the inclination you can read through the Care Act and find out how it helps you with Continuing Healthcare Funding.

As mentioned on the previous page, there is also fast track NHS funding for those whose condition has deteriorated substantially. The funding is supposed to help when someone comes out of hospital with an end-of-life diagnosis. You can find information about this on the NHS Continuing Healthcare Fast-Track Pathway Tool page on the GOV.UK website. If you have been wrongly refused NHS Continuing Healthcare Funding, whether fast-track or standard, you can go to a lawyer (there are quite a few who now specialise in this) and make a retrospective claim. An organisation called Beacon gives free independent advice on NHS Continuing Healthcare Funding which you can find on their website.

NHS funded nursing care
This is for nursing homes only; that is, homes that employ nurses on site. You have to be found not eligible for NHS Continuing Care Funding before you can be considered for NHS Funded Nursing Care. The amount is fixed and is paid directly to the nursing home by the ICB. Your loved one must have a nursing Needs Assessment first. The payments are currently approximately £200-£300 per week. Again, it is worth noting that these payments can affect eligibility for some benefits so just check before you apply to make sure you're not going to lose out on anything.

What you can get for free
There are some services the council has to provide free of charge if you've been assessed as needing help. These services aren't means-tested so it doesn't matter what your income is.

The way to apply is to ask the adult social services team in your area for a 'home assessment'. You can do this by phoning them or going online. Once they have received your application an occupational therapist will come round to visit your relative to assess their needs. If they think a piece of equipment is needed and it costs less than a thousand pounds, the council must provide it free of charge. The sorts of things that are included are small bits of equipment or adaptations, for example, a bath chair or grab rails. If your loved one needs improvements to the heating system and it would negatively affect their medical condition if they didn't have adequate heating then this should also be provided. If the hospital provides any equipment to use once back at home, such as a toilet surround frame, this should also be free.

When A Parent Is An Abuser

What it must be like to care for a parent who abused you when you were a child is hard to imagine. Many care workers seem to assume that the children of the elderly adults they look after have all been much loved and had fairytale childhoods, when this is not the case. To have to do all the things for someone that they didn't do for you must be soul destroying and I don't know how people do it, if indeed they do. Alternatively, trying to take care of an elderly parent who turns into an abuser because of their disease is also a very frightening prospect. Of course, having an abusive personality and having dementia are two different things but having both together can create a dangerous situation. There is a possibility that both are related and that one possible cause of dementia could be trauma in earlier years, whether physical or psychological.

Imagine you have an eighty year old father who has just come out of hospital and you feel you should go and stay in order to look after him. He is refusing to go into a care home or employ carers from an agency. You may feel you have to stay out of a sense of duty. When you arrive your father does nothing but criticise you, shout at you, order you around and tell you that you are worthless. During the worst rages you may have things thrown at you or be so verbally abused that eventually you break down. Psychological abuse includes emotional abuse, control, coercion and intimidation, for example an elderly relative may set you up to be humiliated in front of siblings or other relatives, they may bring up traumatic or uncomfortable childhood experiences or tell lies about you to friends and family. Some parents may try to make you feel guilty when you are not at fault. I have heard of situations where parents accuse their children of hurting them in order to get them into trouble. This could be either because they are hallucinating or just because they are narcissistic and want to be the centre of attention. One parent may accuse the other of being unfaithful or of trying to steal from them or harm them. They may laugh at you when you become upset or say things like, 'You're useless', 'I wish I'd never had you', 'You just want me for my money', 'You're just waiting for me to die,' or the old classic, 'I gave you an education so you'd look after me in my old age'. What a lovely sentiment! To have a child in order to use it for money or as an unpaid carer. What kind of society has as many children as possible in order to use them as servants? Some do, but I have always hoped that ours is not one of them. Potential responses to all this include: 'Tough luck, I'm the best you've got', 'I'm sorry you're upset but since I've done nothing wrong I have no reason to feel guilty' or 'If you speak to me like that again I will walk away'. You could also step away from them or leave the room. Another tactic they may use is to go into 'hostess mode' when talking to another sibling or a carer or doctor. Hostess mode, or 'show timing', as it is also known, is when a person with dementia is able to put on an act of normality in front of certain people, such as medical professionals. This can be exasperating for you as you will have had to give up time to attend appointments and may well feel as if medical staff are going to be completely taken in by your elderly relative's convincing performance. As soon as the person with dementia is once again alone with you they will revert to their usual behaviour and no one will have witnessed it. This is all part of their manipulation of you.

Other family members may react negatively to you removing yourself from the situation but this is really what you need to do in order to protect yourself. Caregiving can be dangerous psychologically and physically for you. Looking after yourself is not selfish! You need help from professionals and you need it as soon as possible. There are many other people going through similar experiences. Remember you are not alone.

Some physically abusive behaviour that parents may display include hitting, kicking, biting, scratching, pulling hair, or using other types of physical force. This is domestic violence and may have started long before your elderly parent actually had dementia. Their goal is to control and manipulate you in order to make themselves feel better and it is extremely hard to extricate yourself from this kind of situation. I have great admiration for survivors of this kind of abuse.

If your elderly relative is in a care home setting then violent behaviour could cause them to be evicted from the home. Dementia can cause mood swings and violent outbursts. A person may seem perfectly fine one minute, then be screaming the next. Researchers think this is probably due to changes in the neurochemistry of the brain with the onset of dementia. There are specialist care homes that do offer one to one care or can cope with violent residents who suffer from dementia using different techniques such as distraction or intervention. These are very expensive however. The only other alternative I have heard of is an elderly mental health ward in a hospital. Some people believe the violent behaviour is a temporary stage of dementia and when people get frailer physically their immobility stops them from being able to be violent. However, this is little comfort to those relatives going through the nightmare of having violent relatives with dementia or to the patients themselves.

It is worth noting that just because someone has dementia it does not mean they can't be subject to criminal proceedings. Courts will take their condition into consideration and look at how it relates to their aggressive or antisocial behaviour but will not necessarily vary their sentencing. Just because someone has dementia it doesn't mean they will be allowed to carry on causing harm to others or themselves.

The Serious Crime Act 2015 created the offence of 'controlling or coercive behaviour in an intimate or family relationship'. It doesn't matter whether the victim and the alleged perpetrator live together or not at the time the behaviour takes place but the behaviour must have caused the victim to fear violence on at least two occasions. The other piece of recent legislation which may be relevant is The Domestic Abuse Act 2021 which came into force in April 2021. This Act created the first statutory definition of domestic abuse and at last prevents the guilty party from cross examining the victim in court which is a very cruel practice. The Act also created the Domestic Abuse Protection Order. To apply for this you can use the online service at RCJ Advice's CourtNav service. You can also call the police. They have the power to serve a Domestic Violence Protection Notice on the perpetrator. When you are in immediate danger it may be hard to reach a phone or to communicate with emergency services. What to do when you have been assaulted and can't speak? If you are in danger and unable to talk on the phone, call 999 and listen to the questions from the operator and, if you can, respond by coughing or tapping on the handset. There are domestic abuse helplines and a list of organisations that can help you on the GOV.UK website.

Dementia can, I found out from talking to other caregivers, cause a complete change in personality, so that even a relative who may have been a wonderful, kind and down to earth person throughout their life may suddenly change and become aggressive and violent. This can be deeply upsetting because you are having negative feelings about someone who has been so supportive of you during their life before dementia and they are suffering from a horrific illness. It's not their fault. But it's not your fault either. It's more than okay to not want to be a carer in this situation. Once caring for a loved one starts to effect your own mental and physical state, it's time to let go and let the professionals deal with it. Once you tell social services you are withdrawing they have a responsibility to care for your elderly relative.

Care Agencies And Other Intruders

In order to obtain care for your loved one you will need to trust an array of people, all of whom will be coming in and out of your home on a daily basis. My own personal experience of care agencies was extremely disappointing. They very rarely turned up on time, which made it difficult to plan anything, least of all my working life. The excuse would always be that it was difficult to get staff or that people were off sick. However, this is not what you are paying for. You are in a situation where you need consistency and reliability. If they are not providing this it may be a good idea to find a better agency. I found the carers themselves extremely variable. Some were really hard working and in fact tried to make up for what the others didn't do, some were rude and aggressive, some were polite and some were wonderful at talking to mum, whereas some spoke to her as if she were a five year old child. Some asked me endless questions, which, when you are looking after someone who is already asking questions all day is the last thing you want. Your elderly relative may resist having carers in his or her house at all. They may refuse to have a bath or shower or have their hair washed by the carers or you. I found dry shampoo was helpful at one stage. I also asked a chiropodist to come round to do mum's feet on a regular basis, although this can become quite expensive. It is worth checking the contract with the care agency to find out exactly what they see as their responsibilities and what they see as yours. I think a care agency should be responsible for personal care such as washing, brushing teeth or getting dressed and that should be included in the contract.

There was one occasion in particular when I felt badly let down by the care agency. It was a normal day at work. I noticed my phone ringing but couldn't take the call. An hour later I looked at my phone again; there were four more missed calls with messages left. I listened to one of them. The care agency; the agency I had employed on mum's behalf to look after mum and give me some respite, were telling me that mum had 'gone missing' and I should call the police and come home immediately. I tried calling back but the 'carer' who had left the message was not answering. I felt bad about leaving work but luckily they were very understanding. I called the police and told them my mother was missing. On your journey as a carer you will find that there are many people; care agencies, nurses, doctors, chiropodists, neighbours and family members, who you thought were your friends and allies who are nothing of the sort and would rather shift the blame onto anyone but themselves. The implication was that I wasn't looking after mum well enough. Why was I letting her go out alone? I rang the care agency and emphasised that I had no control over where my mother went or what she did. I did not have a DoLS (Deprivation Of Liberty Safeguarding Order) and I could hardly stop her from going out or moving around if that was what she wanted to do. They replied that they had entered a safeguarding concern with the local authority and that social services would be getting in touch with me. I returned home feeling scared, upset and confused. But I was relieved to find mum in the kitchen, making a cup of tea and no worse off than she had been in the morning. The main thing was that she was alright. I called the police to say she wasn't missing and then called the neighbours and the care agency. A few days later social services phoned me and said I had been reported to them. The implication was that I wasn't caring for my mother well enough. I wondered whether this had anything to do with the fact that I had raised a complaint with the care agency the week before and had let them know that I would no longer be needing them!

When you choose a care agency make sure you read the contract very carefully, in particular, check how much notice you have to give them when you want to fire them. This is because if you are not happy with the service or they end up being abusive then you want to be able to prevent them coming into your home as quickly as possible. Make sure that you sign the contract with the care agency before they start work and that their contract includes information on their complaints process. If you are unhappy about a care agency there are lots of things you can do. If you feel too intimidated by them to raise a complaint with them there are service regulators you can go to. You have a right to have a camera in your home and you have a right to record in writing how well or badly the care agency are doing their job. They may have a right to raise a safeguarding complaint because an elderly person is vulnerable but you have a right to fight back and raise a safeguarding concern against them too. If you are concerned that the service is not registered or is not coming up to standards you can contact the CQC (Care Quality Commission) in England or if you are living in Wales it is the Care Inspectorate Wales.

Theft and care agencies

In care home settings and private homes theft is unfortunately a common occurrence. It is often perpetrated by the very people who you have trusted to look after your loved one. Theft of jewellery is one of the most common crimes. This is the responsibility of care home and care agency managers who should do an inventory when the person enters the home or starts having care at home and make sure that everything is given back or still there at the end. If a care worker steals from or abuses you or your loved one then that is both a safeguarding and a criminal offence. You can call the police, even if the care worker is an ex police officer. Don't be afraid to call the police and don't be afraid to call the Care Quality Commission. You have a right to do this. You are trying to deal with a deeply distressing situation while feeling emotionally exhausted. You have to look after yourself. Do not feel bad and do not worry that you are negatively affecting the care agency's business, you are in an extremely vulnerable situation and you need to protect yourself and other people in the same situation. You are doing those other vulnerable people a favour. You can complain about a care service by going online to CQC.org. (Care Quality Commission). They inspect thousands of care providers and you can contact them anonymously. Care homes must protect residents from personal threats, financial abuse or from being looked after by unstable and unsuitable staff. A care home or agency must do Criminal Records Bureau checks.

Some people with dementia may find keeping track of their personal possessions a real challenge. They may talk about possessions they owned in the past that they no longer own. That is why property inventories should be kept by care homes in the resident's file. You should always report any lost property. Care staff who are guilty of stealing from residents should be referred to the Independent Safeguarding Authority so that they can be prevented from working with vulnerable adults again. The care home or agency should have disciplinary procedures in place for situations where staff are guilty of theft. Additionally, a care or nursing home should have lockers and safes for keeping valuable items.

Firing the care agency

If the care agency staff are being abusive or disrespectful towards you or your loved one you have every right to sack them. It is a good idea to have an alternative agency to call on to take their place as soon as possible so as to have a smooth transition between one agency and another. More importantly, the care agency you have sacked will probably begrudge your criticism of them and tell social services you are putting your elderly parent at risk if you aren't able to give them the name of another agency you have employed to take over straight away. I called the Citizens Advice Bureau when this happened and they were very helpful and kept my case open so that I could contact them again if I needed to. Once the care agency's notice period has ended make sure you get the locks changed and change any codes for the key safe. It may also help to have cameras in your home or a friendly neighbour who can watch the house to make sure no one is coming in who shouldn't be.

What if they're still coming into your home?

This happened to me and was hugely upsetting and felt like an invasion of privacy. A care agency can't do this if the contract has ended because it is private property. However, during the notice period they could come in even if you ask them not to, in order to ascertain that your elderly relative is safe. This is reasonable provided they are only staying to find this out. If the vulnerable person is safe and well the care worker must leave immediately. So, if an agency worker is being abusive to you or your loved one, or is trying to gain entry to your home when you have told them not to, phone the Citizens Advice Bureau and the police. In my case I had encountered issues with one of the care workers at the agency mum was paying for. I had explicitly asked the agency not to send that particular carer any more. I had phoned them to say this and had also emailed them. However, they kept sending the same person, who came into our home at times when I was at work unbeknown to me. Beware care agencies who are unresponsive and do not act swiftly on your complaints. The only time that someone can enter your home if you ask them not to, other than as stated above, is if they have a court order, are police officers or are from other emergency services (more on this later). You can complain about a police officer by visiting your local police station, calling 101 or filling in an online form which you can find on the Independent Office For Police Conduct website. The powers of the police can be found in the PACE codes of practice. PACE stands for the Police and Criminal Evidence Act 1984. It's a really important code that all police officers must learn when they join the force. It not only regulates the police but is also meant to protect your rights.

Can the police enter your house without a warrant? It depends on the situation. They must first try to find a less intrusive way of achieving their aims. There are hundreds of powers of entry and I am not going to bore you with all of them here but in terms of safeguarding the elderly, if the police believe that an offence is being or is about to be committed they can enter a house to arrest a suspect. They can only do this if they have some evidence that this is a reasonable thing to do, for example, if they hear cries for help or are chasing someone they believe to have committed a crime. They should try to gain your consent first unless it defeats the object of their visit. They don't need notice when entry is needed to save a life or when there's been an accident or emergency but they should tell you why they are entering and what their powers of entry are. If you refuse entry they must document this. If they have visited at a time when no one is home then the police must leave a written notice saying why they visited and it must be left in a place that is easily visible.

Of course in a case of domestic violence, as mentioned in the previous chapter, you may be the victim of abuse at the hands of an elderly relative with dementia and therefore need the assistance of the police. In an emergency, the police have the power to enter and intervene for your safety.

A magistrate's court can give the police power to enter premises if someone has a mental disorder and there is suspected neglect or abuse but a mental health professional must be involved in this process to make sure that the vulnerable person is taken somewhere safe and appropriate. Obviously, in this day and age people are justifiably wary of the police, particularly after police officers in recent years have been found guilty of murder, rape and misuse of their powers. Therefore, if a person tries to stop a police officer coming into their home it may simply be that they have lost trust in authority or are afraid that their loved one will be taken away from them. It may not be a sign of any wrong-doing on their part.

What is a warrant? A search warrant is a written document which allows an investigator to enter a house in search of things or people. They are usually issued by a court after an application from a police officer and they take around three weeks to be issued. Police must always leave a copy of the warrant at the property when they try to gain access. If not, then technically their entry could be unlawful. Also, there will be a time limit on the warrant; it is not open-ended.

There have been many cases of fraudsters pretending to be from the police, care agencies or local authorities. These unscrupulous people go round knocking on the doors of elderly people in order to commit crimes. If a police officer, or someone who says they are, is asking to come into your home you should always get them to identify themselves before you let them in. Ask for details of their local station and phone the number (look this up independently) or call 101, which is the non-urgent number for the police in the UK. You could also ask them to show you photographic ID (although if it's a good fake you may not be able to tell the difference). Bear in mind that a police officer should never ask for your bank details, PIN, computer or passwords. They can only take away your computer or other goods if they have a warrant. They should never communicate with you in an abusive or threatening manner. Just because they have a duty to make safeguarding enquiries does not mean they have free rein to gain access to you or your loved one. Remember it is your home too and you have rights. You cannot be forced out of your home, particularly if an elderly person is dependent on you for care. If there are police officers who have acted aggressively towards you there are specialist law firms that deal with cases against the police and you can look these up online.

Meetings with care agency staff
It is a good idea to make arrangements for regular meetings with the care agency manager. They will often tell you that they are instructing their staff to do certain things but the staff don't listen

and don't read their emails. Do not allow an agency to take over your home or your life. Do not allow any carer to tell you that you should spend more time with your loved one or behave differently towards them; they have absolutely no idea of your relationship and it is not their place to judge you; you will probably already have a very busy life looking after other people such as children, grandchildren or a partner. I found that some of the care agency staff, from the two we used, treated me rather like an inconvenience. Did they listen to what I said? Not really. Did they listen to what the manager said? Apparently not. Some of the carers were excellent but really, if you are paying an agency they should all be of a good standard. Don't think you are without power in this situation. You have a private contract with the care agency. They should be meeting their legal requirements by properly training their staff. In some of the better care and nursing homes, regular relatives' meetings are held. These meetings could be very advantageous to you when you are trying to have your voice heard. If the care or nursing home don't have regular relatives' meetings you could try to set them up yourself. The other residents' relatives would probably be glad of the mutual support and companionship.

When care agencies let you down

It is good to have sourced alternative care agencies in advance if you can. There are also businesses which may be local to your loved one that do cleaning, laundry, accompany people to hospital and prepare and deliver meals. You may be able to have a reciprocal arrangement with a friend in a similar situation so that when one of you is let down by carers the other one fills in. Sometimes it is easier to look after someone else's relative than your own.

I remember trying to go on holiday once when mum had dementia. How dare I? I had phoned the care agency to say I was going on holiday for some respite and asked them politely not to call me but still they hounded me with non-essential calls. Needless to say, I didn't get much respite, just a large hotel bill. Simply saying 'no' will not work with some people! Give the agency a friend's number and tell them to call your friend. Tell your friend to only call you if your loved one is at death's door. Then turn off your phone and let your friend be the only one to know which hotel you're staying in.

Live-in carers

A live-in carer could be right for you if you have a spare room (more than one bathroom is preferable). Via an agency, they cost roughly the same as a care home per week, so around £1,100 per week. There are websites dedicated to helping you compare costs of live-in care and the companies who provide it.

If you hire a live-in carer privately you can expect to pay them around £30,000 a year. Obviously, you will then have to think about the legal obligations of having someone living in your house, such as insurance, occupier's liability (making sure the carer has safe surroundings and is not going to have an accident on the property), making sure that the carer has a fair contract and so on. But it could be a good solution for you and could allow you to gain precious time. You would need to do an enhanced DBS check and get references. A live-in carer you employ privately would not pay rent or bills. You would need to make sure they were familiar with dementia and had relevant training; at the very least first aid training and if your loved one had special medical devices the carer would need to be able to use these competently. You would also be expected to pay for a live-in carer's food and transport including petrol and insurance (they would need to have car insurance that covered them for using their car for work). You would have to arrange regular safety checks for the vehicle they are using. You would have a duty of care in this case. It may be a good idea to get legal advice about how much liability you would have if your employee caused an accident or injury during their employment or if they were the victim of an accident themselves. However, bear in mind that a live-in carer would only be able to take your loved one to hospital in a car if it were a non-emergency situation. Otherwise, an ambulance would have to be called for. Knowing, as we do, the difficulties in obtaining an ambulance in this day and age it may be a good idea to think about private ambulance services if they were required and how to obtain them. There are some private ambulance services who now provide care to a home, for example, if an elderly person has suffered a fall. They can also be used for non-emergency medical transfers but currently it still seems to be the case that if someone has a stroke or a heart attack or needs an emergency transfer because of a life threatening event, an NHS ambulance is still the required form of transport.

Live-in carers have the same rights as any other employees. They need holidays and days off too. You should also consider what might happen if you or your loved one did not get on with them. How would you handle this situation? What would happen if one party wanted to end the contract? How much notice would have to be given? Planning in advance will save you from a myriad of problems in the long run; you want to end up in a situation where the live-in carer takes the stress away from you, not the other way round!

There is also something called 'microcare' but I have so far only seen this term used in Wales. It describes very small businesses, ranging from sole-traders upwards, who offer personalised care services to vulnerable people. These businesses can provide personal care in someone's home or help with going out socially or being taken to medical appointments, for example.

Shared Lives schemes

Also known as 'adult placements', these arrangements are especially for adults with enhanced needs that make living alone more of a challenge. It can be a good solution if your loved one is a social person and they are not ready to move into a care home yet. The Shared Lives Team match two people with similar interests (they can get to know each other before they decide to share living accommodation). The carers are trained and have to be interviewed and have DBS checks. The carer will support the person with care needs while still allowing them to retain their own space and privacy. Some people decide to move in with their shared lives carer, while others just receive visits during the daytime.

There is also a scheme called Homeshare which matches people with spare rooms with people who can offer some support around the house. In return the helper will get affordable accommodation. It can help your loved one stay in their own home for longer. Homeshare UK is a part of Shared Lives Plus and the process of home sharing is overseen by Homeshare UK. You can find out more by looking on the NHS Shared Lives portal or

Shared Lives Plus. However, in my opinion, this set up is unlikely to offer sufficient support for someone with advanced dementia.

What is a Care Plan?

A care plan, also known as a 'support' or 'nursing' care plan, is a document created for someone who is receiving healthcare. Every care home or agency has a different template for a care plan but they include more or less the same things. The care plan, in a nutshell, includes a person's care needs, food and drink requirements, medical history and details of the care and support they will need. This makes it easier for doctors, pharmacists and other health care workers to share important information. Care plans are written after assessing the person's care needs and doing a risk assessment. You and your loved one will be able to read the care plan and be involved in putting it together.

As an addition to this there is a 'treatment escalation plan'. This is a document which gives an outline of a patient's care when they are in emergency situations and they don't have mental capacity to make decisions. It includes recommendations for clinical care in addressing their needs as their health changes and possibly declines. When your loved one enters a care home they, and you, should receive copies of this as well as a booklet which should provide useful information about their care and information about safeguarding.

A House Is Not A Home

What are your rights at home?

Strictly speaking, if you are living in someone else's property and not paying any rent and you don't own any part of it, then you have what is called a 'licence' to be there. You don't have the protection that an ordinary tenant would have. This means that the home owner can ask you to leave if they want to and if you don't go then you are trespassing. However, we all know that with the huge cost of university fees and housing, more and more people are living with their parents and are unable to afford to pay a market rent. Sometimes parents will refuse rent, perhaps because they want their children to stay with them for company. Often all members of a family will club together to keep going financially. If you have a disability or are over sixty your parent can't throw you out. Also, they have no right to use physical violence on you, or to threaten your pets. If you have lived in your home for many years but don't pay rent your parent would still have to give you reasonable notice if they wanted you to leave and you could go to the Citizens Advice Bureau or phone Shelter to get more detailed advice.

If you are paying rent

If you are paying rent then you have rights as a tenant and you can't just be thrown out of the property when your elderly relative wants you to go, even if you are not paying as much as the market rent. They would have to follow a legal process to get you to leave. Additionally, whoever you rent from, your home should be free from hazards to your physical and mental health (including in the garden, on the stairs, in the kitchen etc).

<u>**When you own or part-own the house**</u>
If you have agreed that your elderly parent lives with you then it must be safe for them. You have 'occupiers liability' and a duty of care. It would be just the same if you were living in their house as they would then have liability and would have to make sure you were safe. Obviously, your relative cannot just ask you to leave if you part-own the house or own it outright. If they start behaving aggressively and the reason is because of dementia then social services should be called (see the chapter entitled 'When a parent becomes an abuser').

<u>**How will my home change?**</u>
If you are living with your relative you may find that your home will undergo many changes once they have dementia. Your house may no longer be your home. The care agency will occupy it for many hours a day and then there are the cleaners and the other healthcare professionals such as nurses from the local surgery. It will become part care home and part laundry. Incidentally, due to the disease, many people with dementia find machines intimidating. They may, for example, not want to use a washing machine at all. I think there came a point in my 'carer's journey' when I had to wash everything by hand.

When it comes to changes to your home, the care agency can visit and assess what adaptations may be needed. You may feel this is an intrusion on your personal home life (I did). I once had a healthcare professional come to the house for a routine visit. I got a text while at work to say that she had found a gun in mum's bedroom and was very concerned. Why had I left something so dangerous near mum? I pointed out to her that this was a toy starter pistol that had belonged to my grandfather, not a gun and it did not contain or have any capacity to contain bullets. I received a swift apology!

Alternatively, if you have limited time and a busy schedule you can get a home safety check with an independent consultancy which will cost around £600 and you can find them online; just look up 'care consultants in my area'. The advantage of employing a private consultancy is, of course, that you can simply phone them up and get an appointment which is convenient for you pretty quickly (probably within a week). If you can afford to wait you can apply for a home assessment on the NHS website. They will visit your house and compile a report about the changes that need to be made as your loved one gets older. As mentioned previously, the local council should pay for any adaptations which cost less than one thousand pounds. You may be able to get a grant for something more expensive like a wet room.

Some of the home changes the consultancy suggested to me were as follows: to get rid of all sharp objects, to have a fall alarm, to have the smoke alarm connected to it, to contact the local fire service to request a home fire safety check (this is a free service), to get a GPS tracker which can be worn as a watch or a pendant, to look for trip hazards such as loose carpets or rugs, to check the window and door locks and to install a key safe with a code in case carers or emergency services need to access the home. By the way please don't make the code your loved one's year of birth, there are unscrupulous people out there who go round houses trying to gain access using codes like 1937, 1938 etc. until they find the right number!

If you think your loved one is at the stage where they would be open to using assistive technology you can buy some really useful products on websites like the Alzheimer's Society Shop. They sell products that are specially designed for those with dementia such as safety kettles and cups, sensory puzzles, night lights and so on. You could buy a whiteboard and write a list of important numbers on it so your loved one can easily call for help if they need it. Of course, if you are lucky enough to have a garden you could put a padlock on the doors of sheds and garages as they can contain potentially dangerous items. In terms of electrical safety, you could ask a registered electrician to carry out an inspection and give you advice on electric socket protection. To find an electrician, use a government approved organisation which assesses trades-people who carry out electrical work. If you are going to install a stairlift you should be able to get a free quote and a twelve month warranty. By the way, you can get these removed by the same company that installed them when you no longer have a need for them, the company should do this for free as stairlifts are very cumbersome things to try and remove yourself. Stairlift compan-ies are usually very good at removing them promptly.

Lions Club 'Message In A Bottle' scheme

A 'Message in a Bottle' is a scheme whereby a small bottle containing a person's medical information is kept in their fridge so emergency services can access it quickly. A green sticker can be put somewhere obvious such as on the front door of the house and another one on the fridge so it can be easily located by paramedics. You can find information about how to order this on the Lion's Club website. If you fill in the online form they will send you a bottle with green stickers.

Continence cards

If your loved one suffers from incontinence or similar issues the 'Just Can't Wait Continence Card' might help. It can give access to toilets which are not normally available to the general public and so make going out for a trip much easier. You can find information on the Bladder and Bowel UK website. The card can also be kept on your phone. You can use it in hotels or restaurants even when you are not staying or eating there.

Contacting the DVLA

Strictly speaking a car is outside your home but I thought I would include cars as they can pose problems when dementia is getting worse. You may need to inform the DVLA (DVA in Northern Ireland) and insurance company of your relative's dementia diagnosis so it's good to know where the documents are kept. Some people decide to give up driving voluntarily in the early stages of dementia as they don't feel confident on the roads anymore and in a way this can be a blessing in disguise for you as you won't have to worry about that aspect of their safety.

Blue Badge

Is anyone in your house eligible for a Blue Badge? If so you can put one in the car and use disabled parking bays which will help you to get closer to your destination. This may make things easier for you when you are giving your loved one lifts to dentists, doctors and health centres. You can contact your local council to apply for one.

Transport to and from hospital

On one occasion during Covid, I remember going to hospital with mum. We had arrived by hospital transport for a follow up appointment and having waited three hours, we finally got through to x-ray. We were then told that the hospital minibus we thought was going to pick us up had been delayed but eventually, after another four hours, they arrived and took us back to the care home. I hadn't been able to get a taxi, though I did try calling five different companies. It would have been good to have a back up plan for transport to and from the hospital. I have since found out that there are taxi and carer services that will do this, some taxi services even include specialist wheelchair taxis and some specify that they are dementia friendly. If you look on their websites or give them a ring they will let you know if this is a service they offer. They do tend to be more expensive than standard taxis, particularly if you want your loved one to be accompanied by a carer. The wheelchair taxi service can cost from £6 to £20 one way for a short distance. There are also private ambulance services but to my knowledge they don't currently take patients to and from A & E although they may do in the future. Do check beforehand and be specific about the kind of service you need and the illness you or your loved one has. You should also make sure you call these specialist taxi companies in advance to get a good chance of securing the best vehicle for your loved one's needs.

Installing cameras

Home cameras are a very good idea and you can view them on your phone or your computer at work if your boss is sympathetic to this. (It's well worth talking to your manager at work when you become a carer). You can install CCTV cameras and smart doorbells on your loved one's property since it is in their interests to be safe, although you should try to point cameras away from neighbours' homes and gardens, shared spaces or public streets. Make sure that when you sign the contract with the care agency you include a clause in the contract that says you will be using cameras and how long you will keep the footage for. Keep a copy of the signed contract! Remember to check that the date and time on the camera are correct and visible in case you need to prove theft or negligence on the part of the care agency. Cameras cost as little as £30 online.

Door stickers

These you can order online. They say things like, 'No Cold Callers', 'No Flyers' etc. They can be useful if you are getting a lot of salespeople calling. When people turn up at the door and ask if you'd like to buy something, which they will do even though you have put the sticker on the door, you can simply point to it and calmly close the door, or just not open it in the first place!

The Herbert Protocol

This is a national scheme that helps police find missing people, especially those with dementia. You can download a form from the Metropolitan Police website or your local police website. Fill in the form and attach a photo of your loved one. You can add information about their medication, their address, your mobile number or those of siblings and friends. You should include their physical description, such as height and weight, the language they speak and their favourite places such as churches and libraries. You can keep this at home once you have filled it in and scan it. It should be kept up to date with a recent photograph of the person, so that it can be emailed or given to the police when needed. It is another way of being prepared as, when someone goes missing, you will be under a lot of stress. It also saves time for the police. Before you prepare the form do check your local police website and make sure they have a Herbert Protocol and what their particular system is. Getting this prepared and knowing what to do in advance will help you when it happens.

Protection from fraud, scams and violence

I remember one day coming into the kitchen to find mum looking at the laptop with a puzzled expression on her face. She asked me about an email she had received. When I looked at the email I realised it was a scam but also realised that she did not understand this. This was suddenly very worrying. This was at stage two of the disease. From then on I knew I would have to have access to mum's emails and check them daily. Of course I asked her permission to do this and she gave me that permission. People would also come to the door trying to sell things to her. They would tell her that the roof was in a bad condition and needed to be fixed for an extortionate amount of money, or people would phone up and ask her for information and tell her that she needed to give them her bank details. I had to act very quickly in installing a phone service that allowed her to only receive calls from trusted numbers. This service is usually free or costs very little and I found it worked very effectively once implemented. The other thing you can do is to get a video bell that is connected to your phone so you will get a notification when someone comes to the door. This will be disruptive to your work life but it will probably give you more peace of mind overall. You do not want to find that the £20,000 you thought your parent had put aside for care fees has gone to a scammer.

What should you do if the worst happens and your loved one is scammed? The perpetrators of this kind of offence are committing crimes such as theft or fraud. If this happens do not blame yourself; it is not your fault. It is the fault of the person who is the scammer. You can report fraud and scams to an organisation called Action Fraud; they can give you advice and support straight away. Victim Support is another good organisation to contact. You can click on the section entitled, 'Fraud' on their website. But if someone is in immediate danger, call the police on 999 and contact the bank and tell them what has just happened. If you have access to your relative's bank account you could also use the app to freeze it. There is also an organisation called Think Jessica at www.thinkjessica.com, which gives a lot of useful information and support to victims of scams. Scams can make you feel ashamed and guilty. Remember you and your loved one have done nothing wrong, there is no reason to feel guilty or ashamed, and you are not alone.

Fall alarms

To get a fall alarm you will need to contact a company that sells them and as well as the purchase price they cost about £50 a month. The company you choose will need to come and install them. They can also be linked to GPS trackers. But fall alarms can be a blessing or a curse. Why a curse? They tend to go off even when the wearer hasn't fallen. When the alarm sounds the machine will connect to the company's phone line and an operator will ask your loved one if they are alright; this should help keep them calm. The voice will come from the speaker on the machine which may be a bit confusing for a person with dementia who may not be able to understand where the voice is coming from. If the operator doesn't receive an answer, you will be called and alerted to the fact of the 'fall'. A first responder will then be called. This could be a neighbour or a professional. In my experience it is better to get someone professional to do this. Neighbours can't always be relied on and they may start resenting this use of their time. They may try to make you feel guilty because you have not dropped everything to rush home or they may call you when you are away and have finally managed to get some respite. When this starts happening several times a day, and each time it happens you are worried senseless that your loved one has had a serious injury but nothing has actually occurred, it soon becomes emotionally draining. Your loved one may be a little off balance sometimes and may bang the alarm against a piece of furniture, for example. However, you will also need to think about what you are actually going to be able to do when this happens if you are miles away, at work, looking after children or caring for someone else. Also, a person with dementia may not want to keep the fall alarm on and may keep taking it off and this could become a source of arguments.

GPS watches and pendants

These can help. However, as with fall alarms, your loved one may take the watch or pendant off. They may refuse to wear it. You may then put it in a handbag only to have them take a different bag with them when they go out. Sometimes I have found GPS trackers don't always pinpoint an exact location. Some of them fall off easily and they won't be much good once they run out of power. You will then have to run round the neighbourhood trying to find lost watches and pendants which is not what you want to be spending your time doing. If you decide to give them a try you can buy them from Age UK or Careline. I also bought mum a brightly coloured coat which made her more visible and I let local shopkeepers know who she was and asked them to look out for her. (This does depend on the local community spirit though).

Medication boxes

You can buy these online for about £20 upwards. They may be useful when your loved one starts forgetting whether they took their medication or not. You can lock the medication in the box and give it to them when appropriate, or the carers can do this. You can put a notepad inside the box so that you can make a record of when medicine was last taken. I found these quite useful for keeping track of what had been taken and when.

Blister packs

What are they? A blister pack is just a type of packaging but you will hear it referred to in relation to the medications your loved one takes. 'Does he get his tablets in a blister pack?' pharmacists will ask. The pills inside the pack are organised by time and day so you can easily press out the medication; it just makes it easier to remember what has been taken.

Cleaning

Decluttering an elderly parent's home can seem overwhelming, particularly when they (and possibly you) are still living at home. So it's often best to start with less personal spaces. These might include areas like the garage, kitchen, or laundry room. When mum moved into the care home I started doing basic cleaning and, I'm not going to pretend I was fast; it took me weeks. I started with the kitchen and eventually managed to do mum's room, starting with the bed and carpet then making some space to walk around in so that I could tackle the other areas of the room. Dementia sufferers may also collect pieces of paper and write notes on them in an attempt to try to remember things. Your loved one may want to hang onto these, they may have no mental energy to clear up and may not want anyone else to do it.

This is not their fault but a symptom of the disease. There is a need to have everything stay the same as it gives a sense of comfort and reduces anxiety. It just means you may need a shredder!

One of the problems when a loved one is beginning to suffer with dementia is that they don't want to lose control but they feel that they are. Who can blame them? They won't want to give up control of their home so they may resist every attempt you make to change it. It can be extremely difficult and uncomfortable to contradict them when they have always been the one in charge. But there will be things you need to do to keep the property in good condition such as having gas fire check ups, painting or clearing. This is difficult because you may find yourself involved in constant arguments. A deep clean may be a very good idea but your relative may insist it's not necessary. A house and garden need constant work to stay in good condition. If your loved one won't open the windows this may cause mould to grow which has some frightening health consequences. You will ask them to open the windows, they will constantly refuse. It may be the case that they are scared that a burglar will get in and that is why they refuse. It is understandable; anxiety can get the better of all of us when we're feeling vulnerable. This can be very tough on you though as you are only trying to help with the limited time you have. Your relative may get to a stage where they don't even see that repairs are needed. If you can talk to them before the hoarding gets out of control it will help you later on. You may be able to persuade them to let you make some small changes or let go of certain things. Cleaning could take you hours and may be physically demanding. Depending on your own health and mobility you may or may not be able to do this. If you have to sell or rent the property then check if it's worth doing anything to improve it before you sell it; you don't want to give yourself extra work that's not necessary. If you can't face cleaning the property on your own there are professional cleaning companies out there who will do it for you. However, this can be quite expensive. Ten hours of decluttering by a professional will probably cost around £300. Deep cleaning costs around £15 per hour. Decluttering services can also help you with paperwork after a bereavement. Help with hoarding and cleaning a hoarder's house can run into the thousands; anything from £2,000 upwards. Which brings me onto hoarding.

Hoarding

Because of the risk that hoarded properties can cause, not just to you or your loved one, but to others visiting the property, or even pedestrians just passing by, it's a good idea to give the responsibility to professionals. The build up of items like paper and cardboard causes a fire risk and bacteria caused by food waste can become life threatening. Waste removal companies charge a lot because the process of dealing with these hazards is quite involved. But you will be able to give directions to the company doing the cleaning and let them know which areas to be careful of and which treasured items to look out for. They will declutter and then sanitise. They will also deal with any biohazards present in the property like animal and human waste, food waste and mould. They should then give you proof that this has been done and that there are no further hazards. Although it is expensive it will give you peace of mind and could be necessary for insurance purposes. There are various organisations that can help such as Help for Hoarders. I was lucky that I was able to physically do the cleaning myself. I made a timetable and did a little every day. It took over six months but was well worth it in the end.

On the positive side, you may be the kind of person who enjoys family history (I am one of these people) so I do enjoy looking through old photos and documents, collating them and making sure everything that is worth keeping is well preserved and looked after. There may be family documents or photographs which you will enjoy looking at in future years and perhaps uploading to a website such as Ancestry or Find My Past. Another thing you may like to do is make a booklet about your relative's life, including what they enjoy, who is important to them and so on. This may come in handy with care agencies or in the care home. You can easily create these online and print them out or self publish them. If you are doing the decluttering and have a sibling or siblings you may wish to tell them what you are planning to throw out. If they are not living nearby you can always send them photos of items with captions like, 'Do you want dad's old sombrero he bought in Alicante?' They can then reply with a thumbs up or down.

I found that if it was difficult to say goodbye to something but I knew it was useless and it didn't really have any historical or sentimental value I would take a picture of it and keep the picture rather than the item (this happened to me with a toy camel which I couldn't let go of for decades, needless to say I now have a photo of him on my phone and he lives in a cabin at the local recycling centre where he keeps the staff company). Each generation has its own insecurities caused by the living conditions of the time. Having been through Covid, I am sure that when I get old they will find cupboards full of loo roll and paracetamol in my home!

Decluttering may be made more complicated if your loved one has had a business and has kept records of customers or clients. They may have cabinets up in the loft or in storage elsewhere. It's worth trying to find out where these are kept in advance of any serious memory loss so you can locate them later on and sort through them.

Care Homes – When, Where And How Much?

The first care homes in Britain were built in the tenth century and were called almshouses. 'Alms' means to give compassionately to others. They were funded by the rich who believed they were more likely to get to heaven if they gave generously. The almshouse was followed by the workhouse which aimed to house the 'impotent poor' as they were called but thankfully in the 1700s, a French doctor called Phillipe Pinel promoted a kinder approach, suggesting that people be treated as children in need of care and nurturing, which although dreadfully patronising was at least some improvement.

In the 19th century, dementia was a common reason for admission to a 'mental' or 'lunatic' asylum. The term dementia was used but it meant cognitively impaired in some way and it wasn't necessarily associated with old age. 'Brain congestion', was a widely used term, along with other common labels of the day, such as 'mania', 'melancholia' and 'hysteria'. Sadly, patients were often admitted to asylums as a way of hiding them from the rest of society. An ancestor of mine was admitted to Prestwich Lunatic Asylum for what was described in her medical records as melancholia. Nowadays we would recognise this as depression and there would be no need to institutionalise someone for this. However, people with dementia were often admitted to Prestwich Asylum too. So there was often no distinction between one illness and another. All 'disorders of the mind' as they were called were grouped together. Workhouses, as we all know, were created as deterrents so that people would avoid them. They involved hard labour and no proper medical care. To discourage the 'lazy poor' as opposed to the 'deserving poor' workhouse conditions were so bad that the amount of work a resident would have to do was more than that of a prison inmate. My own ancestor died within a year of going into Prestwich Lunatic Asylum. I can't help thinking that her death would have been due to the bad conditions there. I will not mention any of the archaic treatments that went on in such places as some were quite horrific but it seems there was a shift in about the 1950s when mental health and dementia care seemed to improve. Mental illnesses were still stigmatised but by this time there was a deeper understanding of the brain and the emergence of new psychiatric drugs. Perhaps it was also the recognition of the trauma suffered by people over two world wars or the work of Sigmund Freud and other psychologists that brought the study of the brain and its workings to the forefront of medicine. The NHS began in 1948 and there was a feeling that everyone's health, mental health included, was important.

In the 1980s care homes became big business and many owners made millions out of having them. The number of self-funded care homes increased under the conservatives and these private homes were regulated under The Registered Homes Act 1984 (this has now been replaced by The Care Standards Act of 2000). The Care Standards Act 2000 also introduced regulation for care workers and minimum standards that applied to all types of care homes including local authority homes. Under the Act, all care agencies providing personal care for people in their homes had to be registered and the National Care Standards Commission was set up. This also resulted in care homes implementing proper complaints procedures for residents and their families and offering more choice around health care services and recreational activities.

The Health and Social Care Act of 2008 established The Care Quality Commission (CQC), the body that inspects care homes in England. Recently, more luxury care homes have been built. However, the price tag is way out of the reach of most people, being around £2,000 per week. Many of these large builds offer luxury facilities like salons, spas and cinemas. Some even have their own built-in high streets and shopping centres which I suppose is a plus if you like retail therapy. It is also safer and more sheltered for those who are vulnerable.

Care home or nursing home?

A nursing home is geared towards medical care and they will always have at least one nurse on site. A care home will not have this. A nursing home could be the right option for you if your loved one has recently had an operation or has complex medical needs. However, as always, medical support will be more expensive. Care homes that give dementia support will also be pricier and you will often notice that when you go on a care home cost comparison website they will give a range of fees according to the needs of the potential resident. The average cost of a care home in the UK including one that gives dementia support, is approximately £1,200 per week at the time of writing. It usually goes up every year in April.

In order to find a care home or nursing home you like you can phone up homes in the area, make an appointment and go and have a look round. This will probably take about an hour. There are also websites dedicated to listing care homes in your area and giving information about them, such as what facilities they have, what particular medical conditions they cater for and so on. They should list whether or not they cater for people with dementia.

You will then attend for an assessment to discuss your requirements in more detail, usually with the care home manager. They will ask you to fill in some forms and finally your loved one will be allocated a room and a time to be transported from hospital or house to the care home. Their room should have basic furniture in it already and most care homes will have picture hangers and vases so that you can really personalise the room. Try to look for care homes that have relatives' meetings and a good range of activities for residents, as well as plenty of space for wheelchairs and buggies. I think it's a good idea to have a compliments and complaints box as well as a manager who is easy to communicate with; not one you will have to continually prompt for information.

If your loved one is transferring to the care home from hospital and they've had NHS Continuing Healthcare before leaving hospital, they may be able to get the first six weeks in the care home for free, or if being cared for at home, twenty four hour nursing care for six weeks. They may have to have health evaluations but if they do qualify the NHS will provide the help. I don't remember having any discussions with hospital staff about care homes or financial assistance, much of the time I found that I had to do my own research, which is difficult if you don't know something is there to be searched for. So make sure you ask lots of questions about this when in the hospital and also when the transition to the care home takes place. Care home managers are often good sources of information so don't be afraid to ask what is available and how they can facilitate this. Sometimes funding comes from more than one source, for example, you could get some funding from the NHS and a relative could pay the difference. Or the interest on your loved one's investments could pay part of their care. Obviously, contracts will have to be signed but a Care Quality Commission (CQC) registered home should be above board and accountable.

You are of course free to arrange your own care in a care home. The care home should be registered with the CQC and you can look on their website for more details. If you are paying privately you can set up a direct debit from your loved one's account (as long as you have an LPA for financial affairs) and they will then be able to move in. It's really a question of whether or not the care home has beds available and they can accommodate a potential resident's needs. Most of them are looking for new residents and you should be able to find a care home in a relatively short amount of time although of course it means phoning, emailing and going to visit them. When you visit it should be obvious whether or not they are meeting standards. How does the place smell? Is it easy to get a wheelchair round? What's the food like? You will probably know straight away whether or not your relative would fit in and like living there.

Personally, I found most of the care homes I visited to be really clean and the staff polite and helpful but if you are concerned about an older person being abused or neglected in a professional care setting, for example a care home or by care staff, you can contact the local authority. You can also contact the CQC, or raise the matter with the local safeguarding team. The local authority may start an 'enquiry' which sounds rather intimidating but may simply involve having a conversation with the person at risk, it really depends on the situation and it may be that more than one professional needs to get involved and provide support. An advocate may be helpful if the vulnerable person lacks capacity to fully understand what is going on. Whatever the course of action agreed on it should all be recorded and shared with you.

Is a care home necessary?

A local authority could decide to move someone into a care home against their wishes or their family's wishes but only if someone doesn't have mental capacity and they are at risk because their needs are not being met or they are putting someone else at risk. Any action taken must be in the best interests of the vulnerable person. Sadly, human nature is such that the more vulnerable someone is, the more they get preyed upon. That includes you, so make sure you protect yourself too!

Let's say your loved one has a fall and also has bed sores. When they go into hospital doctors and nurses examine them and are concerned. They think their patient may not be getting enough support at home with moving around or having the appropriate wound care. They recommend that when the patient is discharged they are moved into a care home. Your loved one becomes extremely upset and doesn't want to go into a home. You feel you would miss them too much if they were to leave. Will they be forced to go against their will? How are you going to arrange a care home? If your loved one ends up in a care home but really doesn't want to be there and you feel you can cope on your own at home then get some help from an IMCA (Independent Mental Capacity Advocate). They can help you appeal, even if a Deprivation of Liberty Order or DoLS (which I mentioned in a previous chapter) has already been granted. If that appeal is successful, your loved one could return home as long as you show you can provide the right level of support for them. The support plan could include, for example, assistance with skin care and with eating and drinking. You would have to have a team of care workers to take over when your loved one came home which requires quite a lot of planning. Alternatively, you can ask social services to do a needs assessment and ask for support at home. This will be followed by a financial assessment if you are asking for financial help from the local authority.

Obsessions And Regressions

Dementia is a difficult illness to predict. This makes it more stressful for all parties. Imagine you could predict exactly how the disease was going to affect someone. How useful it would be to know in advance that a particular patient was going to have hallucinations or personality changes. At least you would be able to make some preparations. But the brain is a highly complex organ and we are simply not at the stage of being able to predict exactly what behaviours someone who has dementia will exhibit; it affects everyone differently.

There are supposed to be seven stages of dementia. Sometimes medics divide the stages into three but I prefer the seven stage model as it is more detailed. If you look up the seven stages on the internet you will find charts which will give you the corresponding symptoms although these are not exhaustive. Here's a synopsis:

Stage one - this is when there is no cognitive impairment but the disease has started to make changes to the brain, it is just not very obvious and could be mistaken for another illness or condition.

Stage two – at this stage there is mild cognitive decline so you will see symptoms like forgetfulness and a reluctance to try new things or go to new places.

Stage three - your loved one's forgetfulness becomes more noticeable and they may start repeating the same phrases and forgetting that they have asked the same thing before. They may also start losing things or becoming vague.

Stage four - at this stage your loved one will start having problems managing bank accounts and remembering pin numbers. Sadly, they may become intimidated by technology and other means of communication which was once a source of pleasure. They may not want to cook meals but prefer cold sandwiches, they may start making notes on bits of paper to remind themselves of things and most concerning of all they may start wandering.

Stage five - at stage five, which is classed as moderately severe cognitive decline, your loved one may start becoming very confused about where they are and may forget the names of people they know. Oddly, at the same time as wandering they may also become anxious about going out and may not want to step beyond the boundaries of their own home or even a few rooms. They may start to find the normal activities of daily living very challenging and may stop washing their hair or doing their nails or teeth. They will need help with going to the toilet and getting in and out of bed. Bladder and bowel control will most probably be lost by this stage.

Stage six - a person with dementia at stage six will suffer severe cognitive decline. They will be doubly incontinent and will sleep for most of the day. They may experience delusions, pronounced memory loss, slow movement and frailty, although cruelly this will be very difficult for them to communicate to anyone else. They will need help with most daily activities such as going to the toilet, dressing, washing and so on.

Stage seven - this is the last stage, characterised by severe cognitive decline. It is unlikely your loved one will be able to speak or communicate at all and they will need help with all daily activities. They won't remember people they have known and won't be able to move independently. The brain regulates every system in the body and the effects of dementia vary according to the parts of the brain that are damaged so it is both a physical and mental disease. Aggression or personality change can happen at any time but it is more common in the later stages of dementia. While researching dementia I found some of the videos on YouTube helpful. Many of them gave good advice on how to cope during the different stages of the disease. There were also videos that offered strategies and ideas for dealing with aggressive behaviour. Some patients will be aware that they are losing their memory and will be accepting of it while others will be in denial. It takes a huge amount of self awareness to realise that you are suffering from a condition such as dementia. Just imagine; you are using the brain that is failing you to observe itself and try to work out what is wrong with it. It must be terrifying and lonely.

In terms of the duration of each stage of the disease, you will find these on the internet (each one is supposed to last approximately one to two years) but they aren't clear cut and there is no exact set timescale as everyone is different. This makes for more uncertainty for you but at least there are charts and these days we have some idea of how the illness will progress which is an improvement on past decades!

The symptoms of dementia vary from person to person. Our brains are all unique. For example, some people with the disease will forget everything but the worst times in their lives which they will re-live time and time again. If they have experienced a loss such as the loss of a husband or partner, they will regularly re-live the grief and distress which is a very cruel aspect of the disease and must be emotionally exhausting. Some people with the illness will blame others for everything and this is also a symptom of the illness, not a reflection on the person they are blaming or on themselves. Initially, your loved one may mask very well and even convince medical professionals of how competent they are. As I mentioned earlier, they may go into what is called 'hostess mode' which is when they will appear to be very lucid and well organised when they are with others, particularly doctors, nurses and siblings but will be completely different when they are with you. As the condition worsens you will sadly be proved right. Keep a note of when this happens; often dementia will only be diagnosed when the person is at stage four because it will be so well masked beforehand and there are illnesses and conditions that can be similar to dementia. Remember nobody else knows what you are going through and they don't live with a person with dementia so don't allow them to criticise you or imply that you know nothing about the disease.

What about delusions? Yes, as if it's not hard enough already your loved one may start having delusions that you're not looking after them or that their partner is having an affair or attacking them. They may become paranoid and accuse others of trying to harm them. They may hide under tables because they are afraid that someone is trying to enter the house. Worst of all they may blame you, their caregiver, of doing them wrong. You are probably already feeling guilty for not being able to make them better and here they are accusing you of something else that's not your fault. I know of a few people who have two parents with dementia. This can be incredibly challenging, particularly if they are living together. Arguments can arise and physical aggression is a real possibility between two people with dementia who are living in the same house.

When you first start to realise your loved one is suffering from dementia, it can be unnerving because the person who has always been so logical, in control and meticulous, is suddenly making mistakes. Your natural inclination is to believe your parent because that is what you have been used to for so long. For so many years they have looked after you, been in charge of their children, life and home. They will still be speaking to you in an authoritative tone; the same way they have always spoken to you and everyone else. It is of course not their fault; they are probably going through terrible anxiety and pain inside. They may have been a carer for many other people along the way, including their own parents. You might think, 'perhaps it's me; perhaps I'm wrong and they're right.' It's a very strange situation and may cause you to doubt yourself. This can be very mentally challenging and bring you to the brink of a breakdown. You need support and lots of it. The sooner you get a diagnosis of dementia for your loved one the better. Remember that if your mental or physical health goes downhill you aren't going to be able to help your elderly parent, so looking after yourself is a priority.

Physical manifestations

There are many of these. Often, patients with dementia will scratch their own skin. Sometimes it is an obsessive/compulsive behaviour that is hard to stop. But many times, the scratching is caused by something in the environment. Dementia can also seriously hamper a person's ability to move around. As the disease gets worse, you will need help with lifting and moving your loved one in and out of the bed, chairs and the shower. One person will rarely be enough. If your parent is in their nineties and you are in your seventies then obviously you may have difficulty doing this and will need help! Your doctor, nurse or social worker can give you advice on how to get a transfer belt to help with movement. Buying a back support for yourself is also a good idea. Even if you are just moving a person for short spells of time you still need to take care of your back. Sometimes when you are visiting your loved one in the care home there will be a need to assist them in getting to and from the dining room or toilet. All care homes should have spare wheelchairs to help you do this. Also, if you are planning on taking your loved one outdoors for a while do be aware of temperature changes and make sure they are properly warm as people with dementia will often not be aware of how hot or cold they really are. Should you let someone with dementia sleep all day? This seems to be a common dilemma but allowing a person with dementia to sleep during the day isn't harmful in itself. Care home staff and nurses are usually very aware of issues such as bed sores and constipation which can be caused by being confined to bed and they will try to encourage the person to get up and go to sleep at appropriate times.

Health tests

Having to do constant Covid tests, or any health test for that matter on a loved one with dementia can be uncomfortable. It feels intrusive and as if you are taking on the parenting role again. Asking your loved one to wear a mask is hard too, they may not like them and will continually take them off, not understanding or remembering the risks. Although it is likely that there will be other pandemics in the future, I hope that we will find better ways to deal with the situations they create, particularly with regard to dementia sufferers and their families.

Incidentally, there are some very good books and films that have been written and made recently about how dementia impacts sufferers and their families; The Father (starring Anthony Hopkins) is supposed to be particularly accurate. Other insightful works include: Elizabeth is Missing, Still Alice, The Savages and The Notebook. Personally, I haven't read or watched any of these as I think I would find it too harrowing but I have heard that some of them are really excellent at depicting how dementia feels from the patient's point of view.

When's That Wave Going To Hit? End Of Life, The Will And The Funeral

DNR Orders

A DNR is an order not to resuscitate and is sometimes called a DNAR (do not attempt to resuscitate). A DNR order is a legal document that only a doctor can create that means someone has decided not to have CPR (cardiopulmonary resuscitation) if their heart or breathing stops. This means if someone's heart stops the healthcare team won't try to restart it. It was not a scenario I wanted to think about until a friend told me of her mother's experience. Her mother had not had a DNR order and had been resuscitated with the result that she had regained consciousness with broken ribs and subsequently had a much reduced quality of life. I decided to ask other family members what they thought was the right thing to do and to think about how I would feel in the same situation. Would I want to be resuscitated at that stage of life when there was no chance of a cure and with the possibility of worse pain after revival? Probably not. It is a difficult and very personal decision. Remember there are people you can talk to about this such as members of your religious community if you are religious, friends, family, people who knew your loved one when they had capacity, therapists who deal with end of life scenarios and groups of relatives of dementia patients.

End of life and palliative care

Palliative (comfort) care: This category of care is designed to ease pain for anyone with a serious, long-term illness like dementia. It can be appropriate whether someone is dying or not. End of life care and palliative care are important aspects of healthcare training. 'Person centred care' is a commonly used phrase in healthcare nowadays and is about trying to make patients feel as if they are being treated as individuals; not an easy thing for health workers to do when resources are so stretched but nevertheless desirable.

What is a 'good death'? A 'good death' usually means the dying person was treated with compassion, dignity and respect, in familiar surroundings with people important to them close by. Developing an end of life care plan is a way of making sure your loved one has a comfortable, dignified death. This is not always possible of course if someone dies in A & E. Such situations often happen when you least expect them and can be extremely stressful, especially if treatment is taking place in a very noisy, chaotic ward. If it is obvious that things are taking a turn for the worse, you can discuss this with the doctor on duty and ask if it is possible for your loved one to be moved back to the care home or to their own home. You will then have more control over the environment and be able to make it really comfortable and calming. You may be able to play soothing music, make the room smell of a favourite perfume or give your relative a hand massage. The senses of hearing and smell seem to last even when we are in the final stages of life.

End of life care plans are not easy to make as difficult conversations can arise. An end of life care plan is similar to a normal care plan but with the addition of details such as where the person would prefer to die, what kind of pain management they want to receive at the very end of life, who do they want to have with them when they die and so on. You may remember that your loved one used to go to a particular place of worship, in which case you can contact the religious leader there and ask them to pay a visit. Sometimes care homes will have faith representatives visiting on a regular basis. The care team should have the Advance Directive, Health and Welfare LPA and care plan in the folder at the care home. If your loved one doesn't have an Advance Directive or they can't communicate their wishes to you, a discussion with a health care professional or an end of life doula, for example may help you to work out what they would have wanted (more on end of life doulas shortly). Families don't always agree on these things. If tensions start to surface about the treatment plan you can appoint a mediator. This can be anyone from a family member to a professional mediator (although of course professional mediators will charge). The care plan may have terminology in it which is specialised, such as 'syringe driver', which is a small, portable battery-operated device that delivers medication such as morphine, or a PEG which stands for 'percutaneous endoscopic gastrostomy' and is a tube inserted into the stomach to essentially provide food and water directly.

The way people with dementia die is different from one person to another but there are similarities. Some common signs that someone with dementia is close to the end of life include speaking rarely, being unable to do basic activities like eating or moving to and from bed or changing position. Problems like pressure ulcers can surface and should be brought to the attention of carers and nurses who can reduce pressure on the affected area and make sure that any wounds are looked after to try to prevent infection. After a while a dying person's body shuts down. They can't move much, they don't want to eat or drink, and they lose weight. They often get seriously dehydrated and can find it hard to cough up fluid. Many people with dementia get pneumonia at the end of life. When your loved one suddenly loses weight it can be frightening. You may never have seen them look so frail. Not eating is a result of their body not needing so much energy. They will be likely to be sleeping a lot more. Depending on your loved one's spiritual beliefs, it may be a comfort to them to have the people closest to them visit as well as their spiritual leader, if they have one.

If you have a Lasting Power of Attorney for Health and Welfare you have the right to see your loved one's health records. Usually a care home will keep a folder which contains records of all the medications a person is taking, their care plan, LPAs, hospital visits, eating, drinking and swallowing and so on. If you are concerned that your loved one is not getting enough pain relief you can ask to see the file and get an opinion or second opinion from a doctor or end of life medical team. If you are caring at home you can ask your doctor or hospice nurse to let you have some appropriate medicines on hand for pain or breathing problems. Incidentally, when a person has dementia they can be given what is called 'covert medication' which means that the medication can be hidden in food and drink without their knowledge. Although this sounds a bit furtive the decision is not taken lightly and it must only be done in the best interests of the patient. It can be useful when someone has dementia and may not realise that the tablets they are being offered but are refusing are the same ones they've been taking for the last ten years which have done them a lot of good.

You cannot predict when somebody is going to die. Even doctors can't tell how long someone with advanced dementia has to live and that can make it hard to plan ahead. Don't put your life on hold. This may sound harsh but some people don't want anyone with them when they die. If this is the case and they tell you this don't feel rejected, it can be a natural part of the dying process. It's normal to be tired as your loved one nears death. It takes a lot of time and energy to care for someone with dementia. Tiredness from a lack of sleep and stress can cause burn out. Try to find time for rest. Take care of yourself. Tell your friends and relatives what you need, for example, a few days off at a relative's house, a cooked lunch or dinner, time for you to go to counselling or get some relaxation. Don't be afraid to ask for the support that hospice and palliative care can provide. It's normal to have lots of different emotions while your loved one is dying. I tend to feel sad and angry when I lose someone I love. Don't be afraid to cry, everyone is entitled to! Don't be afraid to cry in public, at the care home or at the funeral parlour, wherever that emotion is going to come out, let it out. Professional carers, medics and funeral staff are used to seeing emotional people every day and some of them may cry with you. They are affected too!

In the later stages of dementia, most people can't speak to or recognise people close to them. This can make saying goodbye hard. It can also be very difficult to find out what they want. You may ask, 'Are you in pain?' 'Where is the pain?' 'What can I do?' And they may not be able to answer you which is upsetting as you don't know what to do for them. It may feel like you've been saying 'goodbye' for years as their dementia has gradually changed them. You may feel relief that their pain has finally come to an end. If this happens, try not to feel guilty; it's a natural reaction. The process of grieving is different for everyone, and you may feel a lot of different emotions. It's normal to feel a sense of emptiness, after all the care of your loved one may have taken up most of your time.

Grief is a strange animal (see Hamlet!). When my father died I remember not being able to stand loud noises or the sound of people laughing. Friends of mine who have lost loved ones have suddenly felt very vulnerable, tired or ill. It can cause you to have intrusive thoughts and images, depression and give you a feeling of being overwhelmed. I have noticed I get chest pain (a pain around my heart) when I suffer from grief. I also tend to see people who I think look like the deceased person when I am out. This is a completely normal response to losing a loved one.

Spiritual distress and worry about life's meaning can ensue after the death of a loved one. There are many therapies that can help such as holistic therapy, music therapy or talk therapy, for example, although there are many more. These can be found online or through care homes or dementia hubs. These therapies can help manage anxiety around the end of life.

Death Doula

Death doulas or 'end of life doulas', as they are sometimes called, are non medical. They can give practical, emotional and spiritual support to a person with a terminal diagnosis. I found having a doula very comforting; it means you have someone to talk to when you need to and someone to accompany you when you visit your loved one. Doulas can come up with some really helpful suggestions to make the last stages of life easier, working in the person's home and in hospices, hospitals and care homes at any point in a patient's illness. A doula can help with advocacy, advance planning, conversations about death and practicalities such as being a point of contact for other services. Many doulas are well informed about the health and social services system. I found just having someone to call up and chat to a great help. See End of Life Doula UK for more information.

Death Cafe

See The Brigitte Trust for more information about these. They are meetings held either in person or online to help people talk openly about death and dying. Death cafes are free and open to anyone and attendees can discuss whatever topics they choose. For example: Do I want to be cremated or buried? How do I talk to my family and friends about death? Why am I afraid of death? How do I plan for death in advance to make it easier? It's very informal and cake and tea are encouraged.

What is a hospice when it's at home?

The word "hospice" derives from the Latin hospitum, meaning hospitality or place of rest and historically it has been a place of protection for the sick. Hospices are designed to make the process of dying as comfortable as possible and are usually for people who are unlikely to live more than six months. There are different types of hospice. They are registered with the CQC and there are over two hundred in the UK. Your GP or hospital doctor can refer someone. A district nurse may also be able to refer you to a 'Hospice at Home' service. Some hospices take self-referrals but the hospice will still need to talk to the person's doctor to find out whether or not they can offer the appropriate level of support. By the way 'hospice care' is a style of care rather than something that takes place in a specific building so it can also be done at home. As mentioned before, if your loved one is at the end of life you may be eligible for emergency funding. This is known as the fast track pathway for urgent CHC funding and can be applied for when an individual's health has deteriorated quickly. The assessment process is a lot quicker than it would normally be. The fast track pathway can enable the person to have end of life care in their own home or in a care home or hospice. A nurse or doctor will usually complete the document which states what the person's healthcare needs are and the urgency of their needs. It's reviewed regularly to make sure it matches the person's needs.

Death

This may seem almost surreal when it finally happens. You may have spent days in the hospital thinking it's going to happen any minute, or weeks jumping every time the phone rings. In a sense it may be a relief to know that your loved one is not in pain any more. On the other hand, it may give you a profound sense of loneliness even if you are surrounded by people. Remember, most people will be sympathetic and understanding, particularly if they have been through the death of a loved one themselves. They will realise you are probably going to feel exhausted and that you will behave differently on some level.

If the death was expected, perhaps due to a terminal illness, you or the care home should contact the GP. If the cause of death is known and from natural causes the doctor will produce the medical cause of death certificate and email it to the registrar or, if there is an issue with the death, to the coroner who will then email their supporting evidence or a certificate to the registrar. The doctor will email the cause of death certificate to the registrar also. The registrar will then produce the death certificate which they will give to you. This rarely seems to happen within five days any more. Don't worry if the coroner is involved. It may not be any cause for concern, they may just need to ask you if you are satisfied that the death occurred in a certain way which you believe was expected. However, it is all quite unsettling, particularly just after the death of a loved one when you are understandably on edge. You may need to take some I.D. with you to the Registrar's Office such as the deceased's medical card, national insurance number, NHS number, marriage certificate or birth certificate. The process will take about an hour. The registrar will ask you lots of questions about how the person died, whether or not you were with them when they died, what their profession was and where they lived. They will fill out the death certificate there and then and hand it to you so you can check to make sure all the details are correct. Once it is perfect they will print it out and give you a copy (or copies, depending on how many you want to buy) and send a 'green form' to the funeral director by email. They will also email you a code you can use for the Tell Us Once service. This service helps by informing government agencies and utility companies that your relative has died so you don't have to tell every individual one by one. It doesn't cover everything unfortunately so you may still find that you have to go through all your loved one's paperwork to ascertain who else needs to be contacted. This could be hard work if they had assets abroad.

It is always upsetting to get letters addressed to your deceased loved one years after they have died. Don't be afraid to send them back; just write 'return to sender' on them and put them in the post box. You can write emails to the company to tell them, if you have time. They will usually be sympathetic and take the person's name off their database. If they don't and it really bothers you get in touch and say that you have a right to rectification (go on the Information Commissioner's Office website to read about this) and you insist that they stop sending you mail.

You can find your nearest Registry Office on the GOV.UK website, usually there's one in every town. You may not be able to get an appointment straight away, it may take about a week but then you will receive an email confirming your appointment and telling you what to bring with you. If your loved one was in a care home, the carers will have already asked you for the name of a funeral director. The care home will try to have the funeral director pick up the body as soon as possible. Funeral directors provide a service any time of day or night to move the deceased to the funeral home. The care home are usually quite good about allowing you to come and pick up your loved one's things within a convenient time frame but it is probably a good idea to do this within three or four days if you can. Once the funeral director has the green form they will be able to arrange the funeral.

If the death was unexpected, you should dial 999 and ask for an ambulance and police immediately. You will be told what to do by the operator. The paramedics may try to carry out resuscitation or will confirm the death. You should try not to touch the area where the person died. If the person died alone the police will make arrangements for the body to be moved by a funeral director who is known to the coroner. If the doctor is unsure about the actual cause of death, even if it was obviously from natural causes, or if the deceased died suddenly and had not seen a doctor during the past fourteen days, they will contact the coroner. It is quite common nowadays for this to be done. The coroner may order a post mortem examination to determine the cause of death and then issue the documents allowing the death to be registered. The deceased's body will be with the funeral director and you should not be charged for the length of time the body has to be held. The funeral director should be able to advise you as to what to expect as they will be dealing with these scenarios all the time. When your elderly relative dies alone a doctor will report the death to a Coroner. This doesn't mean there has been any foul play, it is just the procedure that is followed. The Coroner records who has died, where they died and how.

If an inquest has to be held they will release the body to the family afterwards so that a funeral can take place. Again, you should not be kept hanging around for answers about how long it is going to take. Time frames are dependent on the cause of death but sources seem to suggest that it should happen within six months, if not much sooner. This will delay the funeral at an already very stressful time. This will also delay the probate process which may take up to two years as opposed to one. It is a shame that this has to happen to decent people who have done nothing wrong and simply haven't been with their loved one when they died due to other commitments and normal day to day activities. Again, not your fault, simply the law having to cover as many scenarios as possible and cater to as many people as possible at the same time. If the body is released with no inquest the coroner will send a form to the registrar stating the cause of death and you will be able to proceed with arrangements as normal.

If you were not with the person when they died it is not your fault; you are not expected to be with them all the time and could not possibly have predicted when they were going to die. Many people feel guilty that they weren't around when their parent died. Do not feel guilty. Someone who is near the end of their life will often wait until they are alone to die. There are many reasons for this but mainly it is because they wish to go alone and privately. Someone once told me that people wait until they have seen the last person they want to see and then they pass away. We are all different.

Donation of organs for transplant is not usually possible following a death out of hospital, but donation of tissues may still be possible. This is another reason why it's good to know what is in a person's will before they die. You can let the doctor and funeral director know as it may be that the deceased's body will need to be moved to a hospital rather than a funeral directors.

It may sound insensitive but it is a practical reality that if a death was unexpected or involved some kind of trauma you will need specialist cleaning services to help deal with the room or place where someone has died. There are companies that provide these services in a respectful and discrete way. They can be found online and are often known as 'extreme cleaning services'.

The funeral

'How will I afford the funeral?' You may ask. One option, which can be organised in advance, is to take out a funeral plan if your loved one hasn't already done so. If you have power of attorney this should be an expense which the Office of the Public Guardian would see as allowable to come out of the donor's funds. If in doubt, you can contact the Office of The Public Guardian to check.

In the UK, there is no legal obligation for the next of kin to pay for funeral costs if they can't afford it (being a next of kin doesn't give you, or burden you with, any automatic legal rights, by the way). Most banks will release funds from the deceased's estate just for the funeral. They will usually release about £5,000. This will be paid back later when you obtain probate. However, they will only do this if the deceased has this money in their account. In order to protect yourself remember to always ask the bank before you start taking money out! The account should be frozen when the person dies although there are exceptions. There might also be support available through the Funeral Expenses Payment scheme, which can help with costs if you are on benefits. This can help cover things like burial plot expenses and cremation fees. You will find this on the GOV.UK website.

Funeral insurance and funeral plans

With funeral insurance you pay a monthly premium as opposed to funeral plans where you pay in instalments or in a lump sum up front. The beneficiary named in the policy will get the payout after the insured has passed away but inflation may reduce the value of the cover. With a funeral plan you agree on a price for your funeral at current prices which means you don't have to worry about inflation. You choose the extras you want, such as a celebrant or flowers, for example. This can help take away the stress of funeral planning from those who are left behind. If you choose insurance the payment can be used for more than just your funeral and you don't have to use a specific funeral director, but with a pre-paid Funeral Plan it can only be used for your funeral and you do have to use a specific funeral director.

The more open we can all be about what we want for our funerals the better. The period after a loved one dies is not the easiest of times and removing any guesswork can really help. There are many different types of funeral nowadays. Also be prepared for the fact that your loved one may not have the same idea of a funeral as you. My parents were of different religions and while I felt it important that a burial take place, my parents didn't feel that way.

Many funerals in the UK are still traditional, faith-based services, held in a place of worship and led by a religious official, for example, Catholic, Jewish, Muslim and Zionist. The venue can range from a village church to a large, modern crematorium or a small chapel in a funeral parlour. Prices range from £1,500 to £5,000 upwards depending on what you want. There are many add-ons, from having a hearse come to your house or a choir sing at the funeral. All of these cost extra. The more explicit your loved one has been about their wishes for a funeral the better. More and more people are opting for eco-friendly funerals which include a 'green burial' or cremation. Then there's a humanist ceremony which is non-religious but focuses on celebrating the life of the deceased, or direct cremation: This is a low-cost option where the body is cremated without a funeral service. You can then choose how you want to celebrate your loved one's life afterwards. You could have a church service for example, or a family get together.

Be prepared to choose hymns and photos for the order of service (many funeral services include this in their package). Write your loved one's obituary. If you haven't done so already, choose a funeral home and the venue for the funeral service. To have done this in advance will really help when you are going through an emotionally difficult time. It is no surprise that more people are choosing cremation over burial these days; a burial plot costs from hundreds to thousands of pounds depending on where it is. You will also have to buy a headstone and pay a yearly maintenance fee. You usually arrange the burial plot with the funeral director. Burial plots are not usually sold, but are leased for a set period of time. During the lease headstones can be put up above the grave.

What is Exclusive Right of Burial? Exclusive Right of Burial is the name for the lease of a burial plot for a limited period of time. It means that nobody else can be buried in that particular plot for the duration of the period covered by the lease. Eventually the lease will expire. Usually it lasts between fifty and one hundred years but it can be shorter. After this the lease can be renewed but the owner will have to pay a fee. When the Exclusive Right of Burial has ended, the cemetery owner will try to contact the person named in the lease and any next of kin before digging a new grave in the burial plot.

Did you know that in England and Wales anyone is allowed to attend a funeral? They are. However, they're not allowed to attend the wake if it's at a private residence as that is on private property, unless you invite them of course. Funerals can be difficult family occasions. You may disagree with other family members about the type of funeral you want or about the people you want to invite. Again, getting a funeral plan and talking about it before the event with professionals and family members years before you die is a good idea as it will save a lot of uncertainty and tension when you least want it. At the funeral itself prepare yourself for the relatives who you thought were your best friends in the world and would always be by your side no matter what to not come to the funeral. Also prepare for people to turn up who you thought had already died and/or hated your parent. Feel lucky if no one turns up with a marriage certificate asking what's in the will!

Can I Catch It? Diagnosis And Treatments

<u>How we used to live</u>

Dementia was rare before the twentieth century, presumably because few people lived past eighty. A person would be said to have dementia if they had lost the ability to reason. Pythagoras described old age, which was, in those days, presumed to be sixty three years old onwards, the 'senium'; a time of mental and physical decay until sufferers became once again like infants, a sentiment echoed by Shakespeare in that famous speech from As You Like It. Plato said the elderly should not be in positions that require responsibility! Nowadays we would call this ageist and point out that the older someone gets the more wisdom and life experience they have.

In medieval times people with dementia were often described as 'foolish' and the word 'dementia' was first used. People with the condition were thought to be either unable to tell right from wrong or be deliberately forgetful of the bad deeds they had done in life so as not to be held accountable for them. One of the cruellest consequences of this ignorance was that both men and women with dementia were scapegoats for witch hunters. Older people must have used supernatural means to stay alive, they thought, since most people died in their forties. Any behaviour that could not be understood was interpreted as madness and a result of sinful behaviour.

At the end of the 19th century, Czech psychiatrist Arnold Pick discovered the 'Pick body' which was a tangle of tissue and protein in the brain's frontal lobe. Gradually, throughout the 19th Century doctors began to have a better understanding of what dementia was. The work of German doctor Alois Alzheimer made a significant contribution. He discovered damage in the cerebral cortex of a deceased patient who had suffered memory loss from the age of fifty. Fittingly, this type of dementia was named after him.

In the 1930's the electron microscope was invented and enabled scientists to see the tiniest biological specimens such as insects, cells and bacteria. Using the microscope it became possible to see plaques and tangles in the brain. Then in 1972 English engineer Sir Godfrey Hounsfield invented the CT scanner, (a type of specialised x-ray test) which shows soft tissues and blood vessels in the body. It works on the principle that you can determine what is inside the body by taking x-ray images all the way around it. Hounsfield bravely used himself as a human guinea pig for his prototype head scanner.

Does dementia run in families?

Well, about 1 in 4 people aged 55 years and over has a close birth relative with dementia. It is a complex disease though, caused by many factors, not just your genes. At time of writing, the belief is that you are not bound to get dementia just because you have a parent with it. The one type of dementia that seems likely to be caused by a single gene is frontotemporal dementia. This type of dementia is rare and tends to affect younger people (Pick's disease is one type of frontotemporal dementia). If there's a strong incidence of dementia in your family and you want to know, it might be worth having a test done. You can get a test done on the NHS and 23andMe also do a DNA test that costs around £150. There are genes that are linked to inherited forms of dementia and they can be passed from parent to child. So if you are the kind of person, like me, who prefers to know rather than not, you may be interested in having a DNA test. Many tests also include counselling by phone or in person.

Blood tests are now being developed to diagnose dementia. It is hoped they will be available within the next five years. They will test for the biomarker for Alzheimer's Disease called p-tau217, which can indicate levels of amyloid and tau in the brain. Again, you may not want to know, but if you do, the blood tests could help in preparing you for dementia and therefore minimise its effects on your life and the lives of your family members. There are also some home test kits which measure risk factors for dementia such as blood sugar and vitamin deficiencies. You can find these online. Whether or not they are useful I can't say, but they could give you a positive insight into your health.

Once you know your risk, you will be able to start thinking years ahead about your diet, exercise and finding out about drugs that can slow the disease. You will be able to discuss the ramifications of the disease with family and friends. It is a good idea to factor in the changes that are going to happen not just to your memory but also to your personality as you age. I think anything that can help people plan ahead and give them choices is a good thing.

However, also bear in mind that there are many positive developments in the treatment of dementia. You can reduce your likelihood of getting dementia by doing more, yes, you guessed it, exercise, which improves blood circulation and so of course is good for your brain. Cardiovascular exercise has been found to increase neuron growth and neural network functioning. High blood pressure is a risk factor as is diabetes so if you can, try to give up sugar. (I haven't managed to do this yet so I cannot preach!). A diet full of anti-inflammatory foods, such as a Mediterranean diet, is what you're aiming for.

There are many different drugs being developed that are designed to slow down the advance of dementia. The medications currently available in the UK can help with the symptoms but don't treat the cause. Cholinesterase inhibitors (CIs) improve memory recall for people with dementia and they work by blocking the breakdown of Acetylcholine which is a neurotransmitter (a chemical that helps nerves communicate with each other). You may be more familiar with their brand names: Donepezil, Rivastigmine and Galantamine and may have seen them in your relative's medicine cupboard. Also available are anti-amyloid therapies such as Lecanemab which works by telling the immune system to clear out the build ups of amyloid-beta. There is also a commonly prescribed drug called Memantine which blocks the effects of glutamate. Glutamate is a neurotransmitter which you would think would be a good thing. However, when there is too much glutamate it will damage the nerve cells in the brain. In other words you have to have just the right amount, neither too little, nor too much, for the brain to function optimally.

Dementia can be physically exhausting for the body to cope with so you may find your loved one needs to sleep for many hours a day. The brain produces less melatonin as dementia progresses and that's the hormone which regulates sleeping and waking. Also, because those with dementia aren't as active as they used to be they probably won't get tired when it's night time. Additionally, some medicines that are prescribed for those with dementia actually have a side effect of causing drowsiness, such as anti-depressants, antihistamines and antipsychotics. So don't worry if your loved one sleeps more and more during the day, any of the above could be having this effect.

As we all know medicine is not really an exact science, it is based on observation and the recording of empirical evidence to predict what is likely to happen to anyone's body in the majority of cases. However, one of the current theories is that a protein called amyloid is to blame for Alzheimer's. This protein builds up and damages brain cells. The new drugs coming in over the next five to ten years are designed to remove amyloid protein from the brain. They should at the very least slow down the disease; if they can reverse it, even better but we will have to wait and see. There is also a new drug called Donanemab (different from Lecanemab as it targets larger brain plaques) which is currently being trialled. This, it is hoped, will target what is currently thought to be the cause of dementia; the excess proteins which cause amyloid plaques in the first place. Trials have been promising, showing a reduction in plaque build up, however, some side effects have been noted and more testing is needed. There are so many new drugs coming onto the scene that I can't mention them all here but this fact, in itself, is very positive. Having seen the development of MRI scanning, gene editing and a phenomenal transformation in the understanding and treatment of mental health conditions I am optimistic about the future of dementia treatment.

Other treatments include TENS machines which use electricity to activate a person's nerves. Some scientists believe TENS machines may help decrease pain, but others disagree. Having tried it myself when I had a frozen shoulder I would say it was more of a distraction than anything but I still felt it was more beneficial than not.

Therapists may also use cognitive stimulation therapy (CST) to improve certain aspects of dementia such as memory, problem solving skills, communication abilities and anxiety. This therapy involves games, puzzles and practical activities like baking or gardening. Many care homes now include daily activities such as these in their schedules which, at the very least, are social and enjoyable.

In care homes residents who love animals will happily group around them and this leads to enhanced social interaction between them. Animals do a fantastic job of uniting people and providing love and companionship. Also music and dance, as well as performances that are given by local groups, physiotherapy and water-based exercise seem to be very beneficial. Occupational therapists help people with dementia to improve their ability to complete activities or tasks by simplifying daily activities thus allowing them to retain their independence for longer. There are many types of gentle exercise, yoga or relaxation classes that take place in care homes on a weekly basis and these can help increase confidence where it has been lost as well as improving coordination. On a one to one basis, talk therapy, or psychotherapy, can help people talk through their experiences with a mental health professional. Talk therapy can help people with dementia recognise and address behaviours and emotions that are causing them anxiety.

Reminiscence Therapy can be helpful for those living with dementia. What is reminiscence therapy? It is simply a type of psychotherapy that involves recalling past events. A person with dementia may well be able to remember things that happened during their youth, but find it hard to recall what they did half an hour ago. It seems to be the consensus among researchers that older memories are still stored in the brain even until the late stages of the disease. Reminiscence therapy tries to tap into these stored memories. It can be as simple as sitting down in a group and talking about things people used to do at school, for example, or games you used to play. TV programmes about going back in time to previous decades are lots of fun to watch. What were your favourite sweets, toys and pastimes? Talking about these things can give a great deal of comfort and happiness to people with dementia. Foods you used to eat, smells, such as old fashioned soaps, or childhood songs can all be part of the therapy. When a person with dementia listens to songs of a certain era this can stimulate the brain and that person will be able to talk about their experiences at that time in their life. If however they were simply asked straight questions about these experiences they may not be able to answer. This can have a very positive effect on your loved one and bring back some of the self-esteem they have lost in their struggle against the disease.

When someone has dementia, memories seem to be lost in reverse order so that the ones that were made many years ago remain for longer. Short-term memory loss is partly due to the depletion of neurotransmitters (the neurons that allow one nerve cell to 'talk to' another) and also partly due to the deterioration of the hippocampus, which is the area of the brain where memories are stored. The hippocampus shrinks during the disease, so that information that enters the brain is not retained. Of course it's the positive experiences we want to remember. We don't want to become fixated on negative or painful memories but unfortunately it seems we cannot choose the ones we want to keep and the ones we want to forget.

In terms of the general care of the elderly, vaccines are being developed to help prevent Urinary Tract Infections (UTIs). These could help because many elderly people with dementia suffer with Urinary Tract Infections and these illnesses have symptoms such as vagueness, tiredness, confusion which will make it appear that the dementia is getting worse.

Then there's I.T. Don't get me wrong, I love the internet and I think it's made some really positive changes to society, including the many support groups that exist for carers. However, the older population may have fewer digital literacy skills and people with dementia often need a lot of support in accessing zoom meetings or face time calls, for example. Again, this may cause more unwelcome work for you when you come home after a long day or are visiting your loved one. First of all, you will have to convince them it is a good idea and then you will have to help them turn on the laptop or tablet, help them find and input the password, use the mouse or finger pad and so on; you get what I mean, after an hour of exasperation you will be wanting to write the emails yourself and send them. Some people with dementia have a real fear of technology and won't use computers, the internet or television. Some absolutely hate having electricity or heating left on. You may find yourself quite limited in how much electricity, water and gas you can use when you are living or staying with a person with dementia.

Many people living in sheltered accommodation or a care home are now using smart technology to facilitate their own care, using it to order the weekly shop, play music or tell us when they are getting out of bed. Some of these technologies can save us time and effort but they can also invade our privacy and prevent us from trying to do things for ourselves. Will you and I want this technology to be used in our own care? If so, to what extent? Will it be a case of picking and choosing them in advance and putting this into a living will? After all, not everyone wants to use robots in their care. Not all robots are what they seem! They come in many guises. Some robots can help lift people with mobility issues or detect falls, feed people and help them use the toilet. These robots can save carers, including care home staff, from the physical demands of caring such as lifting, carrying and transporting residents. However, these machines do need looking after themselves and will at some point inevitably break down. Others are aimed at entertaining older people, though whether this goes beyond simple novelty value is debatable. Some robots are designed to look like cats, dogs or other pets; they will wriggle, flip and purr. These can work quite well in providing comfort to someone with dementia, particularly as distractions or talking points. However, some people with dementia can become overly attached to these toys and others can ignore them completely. The robots don't seem to help with repetitive behaviour patterns and can end up causing more work for care staff as they have to be looked after, sanitised and stored.

What I experienced with robot pets was that mum did like the purring cat. In terms of communication technologies she loved to speak to family members and friends on WhatsApp as long as this was set up for her. She also loved music, so when I visited I used to play classical music for her on my mobile phone. I do believe there is a place for machines that help with lifting, carrying and monitoring but when it comes to entertainment I'm not sure robots are the whole answer. I personally find that the 'cuter' the developers try to make robots look the more creepy the result; particularly the ones with human grown skin! Certain horror movies come to mind!

Face to face interaction surely can't be replaced by a machine. Humans need to connect with other humans who have lived through histories such as their own or at least those who can empathise with their pain. The other point to be made is that technology is not reliable. It doesn't always work and let's face it, in most computer programmes there is a 'glitch' of one kind or another which only a very few people involved in its design and writing will be aware of.

<u>What are memory clinics?</u>

You will need to ask a GP to refer your loved one to a memory clinic. Unfortunately, most GPs are not specialists in dementia and they don't have the time or resources to spend on it. This can mean that they don't diagnose the disease early enough (your loved one may be able to mask their decline very cleverly too) and this can lead to lost time when you could have made plans or obtained medications that slowed down the progression of the disease. In memory clinics in the UK you will find specialists such as psychologists, geriatricians (doctors for the elderly) and nurses who are experts in dementia. Your loved one will be offered a series of tests to check their ability to remember and retain information. It's important to let them know that they don't have to get all the answers right and there's no pressure; it's not an exam! Your relative will also be asked to supply blood and urine samples and they may be offered a CAT scan (computerised axial tomography) which takes x-ray images of the brain, or an MRI (magnetic resonance imaging) scan which can show the damage caused by dementia. If the results of those scans are uncertain then a SPECT scan or a PET (brain positron emission tomography) scan can be more accurate. PET scans are supposed to give slightly better contrast and detail than other scans. x-rays, CAT scans and PET scans do carry a slight risk of radiation but MRIs don't. An EEG uses electroencephalogram imaging to record electrical activity within the brain. This is completely painless. These can help medical professionals to identify brain shrinkage or other anomalies. You can attend these tests with your loved one. If claustrophobia is an issue there are MRI machines which can take images with the patient standing up or ones which are not enclosed. Music can also be played to the patient's choice when having these scans done in order to aid relaxation.

Why is a memory clinic better than a GP?

Unlike a GP, the memory clinic can focus specifically on memory issues, with staff who are specially trained in dementia diagnosis and care. To get a definite diagnosis of dementia the clinic may have to carry out a wide range of tests which the GP probably has neither the time nor the skills to carry out, that is why a memory clinic is preferable. Staff working in memory clinics are trained in understanding dementia and may also be able to identify which stage of dementia the patient has reached.

After visiting the memory clinic your relative may either be asked to come back in a few months for more tests or they may get a diagnosis. Partners, family members or carers are all welcome to attend appointments too. Since there are different forms of dementia such as Alzheimer's, Pick's disease and Dementia with Lewy Bodies you will be given information specific to the type of dementia your loved one has. You will be given telephone and contact details to access further information and support services. Monitoring will continue as will medication reviews. The GP will be notified and you will get a letter giving the diagnosis which may help you obtain benefits and funding for your loved one.

Admiral nurses

They really should be called 'Admirable Nurses'. There are approximately five hundred in the UK currently. If only there were more! One of the problems I encountered on my 'carer's journey' was trying to find carers or nurses who were specifically qualified and experienced in dementia care. It was relatively straightforward to find care agencies but not specifically dementia carers. Admiral Nurses are specialist dementia nurses who have already qualified as registered nurses. They have then gone into a job where they have gained experience of dementia. Every Admiral Nurse gets support and professional development through the Dementia UK Admiral Nurse Academy. Some nursing and care homes also run courses specifically in dementia care in order to support their staff and enhance their professional knowledge.

How We Will Live

In the future we will live with a greater understanding of dementia. Eventually there will be a cure or ways to manage the disease so effectively that it no longer devastates lives to such an extent. We will create manifestos, frameworks for research and health pathways to improve the quality of care for those with the disease. New financial products will enable people to plan for their future care without being left penniless in later life and scientific inventions will allow people to move and communicate more easily. How will we do all this? With huge effort, perseverance and collective innovation. It will not be easy. But it will happen because people are living longer lives. The greater the number of people who suffer the higher the need and change will be necessary.

It was only a century ago that we first began to understand dementia. Since then there has been a huge transformation in the care of the elderly. I am optimistic that in another fifty years time dementia will be re-defined as a disease which, though it has to be managed, can be vastly improved by new drugs and is not the merciless killer it is today. The families of those with dementia are currently lacking the help, care and funding they desperately need, becoming the second patients no one sees. This, I hope will be addressed by the government sooner rather than later.

Nowadays, more and more people in the public eye are announcing that they have dementia which has greatly improved public awareness. The rise of social media has helped too, with relatives getting together in online groups to support each other and raise funds for research. Medical communities all over the world are uniting to share their experiences and ideas; Join Dementia Research and Dementia Research UK are two such organisations.

I hope this book has provided you with some useful information that will help you while you are going through the challenging process of looking after an elderly parent with dementia. I hope it gives you some ammunition against those who would try to diminish the incredible job you are doing. Do not listen to them, be proud of yourself. Even if no one tells you what a kind, patient and wonderful human being you are you must say it to yourself again and again. Your hard work deserves proper recognition. And remember to care for yourself first because if you don't you can't look after anyone else!

*****

End

www.ingramcontent.com/pod-product-compliance
Lightning Source LLC
Chambersburg PA
CBHW071220260726